Publisher's Cataloging in Publication Data

1 - Zimmerman, Julie

2 - The Diagnosis and Misdiagnosis of Back Pain

3 - Bibliography, Appendix B
   Includes Index

4 - Backache
   Chronic pain
   Health, back care
   Medical self - care
   Medical treatment of chronic back pain
   Self - care, health
   Treatment of chronic back pain

Library of Congress Catalog Card Number 90 - 85649

ISBN 1 - 879418 - 02 - 9

Dedication

To Susan, Lloyd and all the other health professionals who join their chronic pain patients in the search for answers

and

To Sandy, Barbara and all the other friends and family members who respect the decision to end the search

Back Pain

Lumbar spasm.
Clenching of teeth around the spine.
It can come on suddenly, with
Devastating clarity, not easily confused
With other pronunciations.

Everything grinds to a halt.
A new consciousness of muscular
Fraility develops instantly and never
Completely resolves. Immobility
Is memorized like a prayer.

And one recovers, as in learning to love again
One almost inconceivably small step
At a time.

Jeremy Nobel, MD

The Diagnosis and Misdiagnosis of Back Pain

Table of Contents

Author's Preface

When I began the search to find a cure for the debilitating back pain that was disrupting my life, I visited my family doctor, an orthopedic surgeon, a neurologist, a neurosurgeon, a rheumatologist, two osteopaths, an acupuncturist and two physical therapists. I tried a corset, acupuncture and the acupuncture diet, manipulation, various medications, bedrest, ultrasound, massage therapy, exercise programs, posture training, foot orthotics and positive thinking. I was advised to base my activity level on the pain and advised to ignore the pain. I was told that I should turn the pain over to God, that I should let myself get well and that my physical problem was a direct result of spiritual negativity. Friends insisted that osteopathy is the one answer, that acupuncture is the one answer and that chiropractic is the one answer. Diagnoses considered included muscle strain, degenerative disk disease, lupus (SLE), rheumatoid arthritis, somatic dysfunction, multiple sclerosis, prolapsed disks, piriformis syndrome and sacro-iliac joint dysfunction. My official diagnosis remains "low back pain".

One of the brightest days in the months of medical appointments and trial treatment was the day my family doctor, husband and I had a conference; we decided that the search for a diagnosis and cure had gone on long enough, that I have a disability which is probably permanent and that it was finally time to get on with my life. It was distressing to give up my career as a physical therapist, a vocation that had absorbed and defined me for years, but it was also an enormous relief to let go of the commitments I could no longer honor.

Chronic pain is with me daily, straining my physical and emotional resources. There is a struggle to maintain self-esteem, but also the emergence of new interests and new horizons. My back pain hasn't diminished in the years since its onset, but I consider myself to be a happy, productive person; it was impossible to be either when my only goal was to resume my former pain-free life. Now I can say "I'm fine!" and mean it.

While searching for answers to my own condition and in my professional research and experience, I have learned how controversial and complicated back pain is. My hope is that *The Diagnosis and Misdiagnosis of Back Pain* can help those of you with acute, chronic or recurrent back pain find the ways to minimize your pain and proceed with your lives.

Introduction

"We are spending too much on treatments that are not proven and on diseases that aren't actually there." Charles Federspiel, PhD[6]

200 million of 250 million Americans will have back trouble before age 50;[1] in people younger than 45 it is the most frequent cause of disability. Back pain is the nation's most common musculoskeletal complaint, with 7 million disabled annually.[25] For 10 percent, or 20 million, the symptoms will become chronic. Back pain, the most expensive benign condition in America, costs up to $80 billion/year in lost wages and productivity,[2] plus many billions more in medical costs, disability claims, lawsuits and related expenses; no other affliction even comes close. Back problems are second only to upper respiratory infections for causing missed work and visits to the family doctor; they are responsible for the largest number of workers' compensation claims and up to 32 percent of disability payments.[25]

The phenomenal scope of this problem should mean that it is well understood. Unfortunately, the controversy surrounding the diagnosis and treatment of back pain proves otherwise. People with back pain frequently receive a variety of diagnoses, misdiagnoses or no diagnosis; finding the right treatment is often a matter of luck. Back pain may continue for months or years despite patients' best efforts and those of their heath care providers.

Diagnosis

"Early, accurate diagnosis is not absolutely essential." Mark Horwich, M.D.[16]
"The cause of chronic pain is a lack of diagnosis; truly effective, relieving treatment is unlikely without a diagnosis." William Wyatt, D.O. [34]

A patient who consults a GP, chiropractor, orthopedic surgeon, osteopath and alternative healer may get five different opinions as to the cause of his back pain. Each health practitioner seems to have a different explanation for a patient's symptoms. Many patients never receive a specific diagnosis and are classified as suffering from "low back syndrome".[31] The majority will never know the true underlying cause of their pain.[26] In fact, few back injuries can be traced to anatomical disorders and no medical test or examination technique can say what actually caused them.[22,30]

Although the principle obligation of a health care professional is to diagnose and treat pathology, there is often little to go on but the patient's report of pain. Health practitioners who treat back pain base treatment on their individualized views of what causes it and in which spinal structures the pain originates; the variation of opinions is staggering!

- *"Trauma is the most frequent cause of back pain, the main reason being that people are in poor physical condition."*[3]
- *"80 percent of back pain is caused by weak or tense muscles."*[33]
- *"50-70 percent of chronic symptoms are psychological in origin."*[5-A]
- *"The majority of lower-back pain actually originates in the sacral ligaments."*[8]
- *"An extremely high percentage of patients with pain have fascial problems."*[7]
- *"The majority of chronic disabling low back pain is from degenerative changes."*[17]
- *"Most neck, shoulder and back pain is due to Tension Myositis Syndrome."*[29]
- *"In 50 percent or more of back pain patients, the facet joint is the site of dysfunction."*[5-B]
- *"Chronic pain is caused by chronic guilt; back problems are due to a lack of feeling supported."*[15]
- *"Chronic sprain is probably the most common low back problem."*[21]
- *"Functional disorders of the musculoskeletal system called somatic dysfunctions are responsible for most (95 percent) back pain."*[4]
- *"90-95 percent of back pain is due to disks."*[5-C]
- *"Vertebral subluxations are found in every sick, malfunctioning body."*[20]
- *"Improper diet and lifestyle are the root of most of our medical problems."*[18]
- And from a British newspaper, *"There is a well-proven relationship between the number of cigarettes smoked and the likelihood the individual will have back problems."*

Obviously, the health care profession does not have a firm grasp on the condition which affects 80 percent of Americans. This is frightening for the person with back pain who wants to know immediately and with certainty

'What's wrong?' 'How serious is it?,' 'Will it get worse?,' and 'What do I do?' Most people assume that curative treatment can't begin until a health problem is accurately diagnosed. In the field of back pain, it is commonplace for treatment to be prescribed without a diagnosis or with a misdiagnosis.

Treatment

"Researchers say there's no clear-cut advantage of one kind of treatment over another." David Zinman [35]
"The vast majority of approaches to treating back pain patients have been found to be no better than no treatment at all." James McGavin, PT [24]

Given the lack of agreement concerning the diagnosis of back pain, it is not surprising that treatment for the condition is equally controversial. Treatment is often based on the philosophy and training of the practitioner rather than the patient's symptoms. Regardless of the treatment approach, 60-80 percent recover from an acute low back pain episode in three days to three weeks;[9] 90 percent recover within two months.[10] Most back aches get better despite treatment rather than because of it. When spontaneous recovery and medical intervention fail, back pain becomes chronic. Treatment continues, but it is often expensive, inappropriate and prescribed in response to the patient's pain level, not to address known pathology. The desperate wish for a quick fix also encourages non-conventional approaches which may be harmful. Many patients shop around and try, in the words of one neurosurgeon, "injections, stimulators, mechanical devices, and Rolfing, none of which can possibly have any curative effect."[14]

Although an army of "experts" claim to have found the answer for "most" back pain patients, this field has a dismal percentage of cure. Claims made concerning the success of various treatments cannot be taken at face value; if the following statements were all true, one would be at a loss to understand why so many Americans suffer from recurrent or chronic back pain.

- *"I haven't seen any techniques that are so effective in reducing pain and restoring function as myofascial release."*[7]
- *"Mobilization and manipulation studies claim an 80 percent success rate."*[11]
- *"80 percent of low back pain patients get immediate relief with epidural blocks."*[32]

- *"In one study, the McKenzie approach revealed that 97 percent of patients improved over one week of treatment."*[24]
- *"With Meridian Therapy 40 percent were still free of complaints after one year and 30 percent were better."*[12]
- *"With microcurrent therapy, 95 percent of patients got pain relief and 82 percent were pain free within 10 treatments."*[27]
- *"90 percent of patients diagnosed with sacroiliac joint dysfunction without secondary factors obtained significant relief with manipulation."*[24]
- *"Radiofrequency facet denervation is more than 70 percent effective."*[28]
- *"95 percent were better or cured with manipulation under anesthesia preceded by a full eclectic regimen."*[19]
- *"In the YMCA's exercise program, 80 percent improve and 31 percent have pain completely eliminated."*[33]
- *"70-80 percent of those carefully screened for radicular symptoms benefit from surgery."*[9]

Although every technique helps some people with back pain, nothing works for everyone. Practitioners who diagnose the same problem and prescribe the same treatment regime for every patient don't help the majority of their patients. The onus is often on the patient to believe in a treatment in order for it to work, implying that those without optimistic attitudes will undermine the healer's efforts. However, it is unfair to expect people searching for relief to get their hopes up again and again. Practitioners of a specific philosophy shouldn't demand total commitment from a patient, but rather an open mind. The test of a treatment's success is what works in the long run.

Given the difficulty of receiving a firm diagnosis and the controversy surrounding the treatment of back pain, patients may despair of ever being pain-free. Fortunately, the people whose back pain signals a potentially serious disease have a good chance of being accurately diagnosed and effectively treated. The other 85-90 percent[6,13] are usually diagnosed with "low back syndrome" or with one of the conditions which falls into this category. These syndromes can be extraordinarily painful and limiting, but are not life-threatening. To provide the best chance for permanent pain relief and to avoid having the condition become chronic, it is crucial for patients to be evaluated by a professional who can relate specific symptoms to specific syndromes and then apply the appropriate therapy. Even if the primary pathology cannot be identified, treatment of symptoms can provide short-term relief. The response to symptomatic treatment may then further pinpoint the structures involved. The long-term goal is for function to improve and pain to decrease even if the specific origin of the problem is unknown.

The Diagnosis and Misdiagnosis of Back Pain attempts to sort through the confusion of advice and promises, terminology and treatments that surround this subject. It explains the rationale behind the various diagnoses and therapies, giving individuals with back pain the knowledge that will let them make appropriate choices when looking for help. What works to the patient's advantage in the diagnostic stage is to be as informed as possible about backs and what can happen to them. Being knowledgeable about what they might be told is wrong helps patients ask pertinent questions, understand the answers and make informed decisions in their own best interest.

PART 1 looks at the normal back, at the training and philosophy of health professionals and explains the diagnostic process. PART 2 provides an in depth examination of the conditions which are classified as "low back syndromes" – their pathology, symptons, diagnostic rationale and treatments. When patients are **accurately** diagnosed with one of these conditions, (ruptured disk, muscle strain, degenerative disease of the spine, etc.), it gives patient and doctor clear guidelines for appropriate intervention. The final chapter, "Author's Recommendations," offers suggestions appropriate for everyone with back pain.

Using *The Diagnosis and Misdiagnosis of Back Pain*

1) The information presented is based on the writings and research of practitioners in the field of back pain. Given the considerable controversy in this area, an attempt has been made to discuss opposing theories objectively and fairly.

2) In keeping with the attempt to present information objectively, the book is written in the third person. The exception is in sections which offer specific recommendations to "you," the person with back pain.

3) Certain sections in the book provide in depth or technical information on specific topics. These are boxed so that readers not interested in such

detail can easily continue with the basic text.

4) For those unfamiliar with anatomical terms, the first chapter, "The Normal Back," explains the normal anatomy and movement of the spine. A complete glossary is included in Appendix A.

5) At the end of every chapter is a summary or overview of the information in that chapter, titled "Key Points."

6) Footnotes throughout the text refer to the numbered resources listed alphabetically at the end of each chapter. A complete bibliography is included in Appendix B.

7) People with acute back pain are referred to as "patients" during the diagnostic process and while receiving professional treatment. When a person's pain becomes chronic, the "patient" designation is no longer appropriate. In this book, people are referred to as "patients" only in the context of diagnosis and treatment.

8) *The Diagnosis and Misdiagnosis of Back Pain* is written for the person with back pain, but is also appropriate for the health practitioner who treats back pain patients. Chapter 14 contains "Recommendations for Health Professionals".

Disclaimer

The purpose of *The Diagnosis and Misdiagnosis of Back Pain* is to provide information regarding the diagnosis of back pain and the recommended treatments for specific diagnoses. It should be used as a general guide and readers should tailor all information to their individual circumstances. **This book is in no way meant to take the place of an individualized evaluation and treatment plan from a qualified health professional.**

The author and Biddle Publishing Company have neither liability nor responsibility to any person with respect to any injury alleged to be caused directly or indirectly by the information contained in this book. If the reader does not wish to be bound by the above, the book may be returned to the publisher for a full refund.

Footnotes

1 Edward Abraham, *Freedom from Back Pain*
2 Henry Allen, "That Back's Gotta Come Out"
3 American Medical Association, *Book of Back Care*

Introduction

PART 1 - THE DIAGNOSTIC PROCESS

Chapter 1 - The Normal Back

Normal Anatomy of the Spine

"The thigh bone's connected to the hip bone, the hip bone's connected to the back bone, the back bone's connected to the neck bone, now hear the word of the Lord!" Source Unknown

"The back" functions as a single unit, but it is a complex structure composed of bones, joints, disks, muscles, ligaments, a spinal cord, nerve roots and all their connective and surrounding tissues. The back is shaped and supported by individual bony segments, the **vertebrae**; together they make up the vertebral or **spinal column**. The spinal column has four built-in curves, two concavities ("lordoses") of the low back and neck, and two convexities ("kyphoses") of the upper back and sacrum. These allow energy-efficient postural balance and serve a shock-absorbing role for the body. The spinal column is divided into five sections: the seven **cervical**, twelve **thoracic** and five **lumbar vertebrae** are separate bones, while the five sacral vertebrae are fused into one bone, the **sacrum**. The **coccyx**, or tailbone, is also one fused entity. [see Figure 1-1]

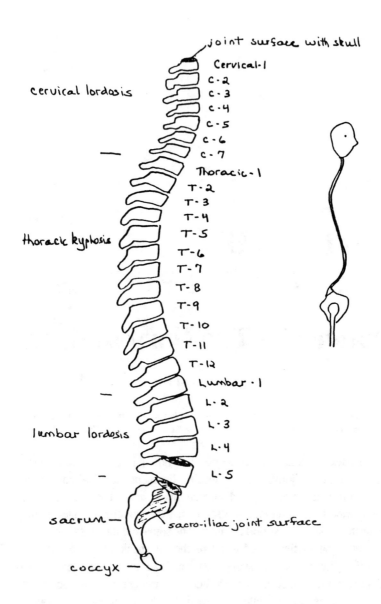

joint surface with skull

Cervical-1
c-2
cervical lordosis
c-3
c-4
c-5
c-6
c-7
Thoracic-1
T-2
T-3
T-4
T-5
thoracic kyphosis
T-6
T-7
T-8
T-9
T-10
T-11
T-12
Lumbar-1
L-2
L-3
lumbar lordosis
L-4
L-5
sacrum —
sacro-iliac joint surface
coccyx —

Figure 1-1. The spinal column, side view.

The spinal column is joined at the sacrum to the **pelvis**; this large bone is a ring composed of three sections (ilium, ischium and pubis). The sacro-iliac joints join the ilia of the pelvis to the sacrum; the pubic bones are connected anteriorly by strong fibrous tissue (the "pubic symphysis"). [see Figure 1-2]

Structures Joining Vertebra to Vertebra

(1) Intervertebral **disks** sit between the bodies of the vertebrae and provide cushioning and shock absorption; they have a tough fibrous outer ring (the "annulus fibrosis") and soft gelatin-like center (the "nucleus pul-posis"). [see Figures 1-3 & 1-5]

(2) Each vertebra has seven bony projections or prominences – a spinous process posteriorly, two transverse processes laterally and four articular processes which extend up or down. [see Figures 1-4 & 1-5] **Facet joints** link the two superior articular processes of one vertebra to the two inferior articular processes of the vertebra above it. [see Figures 1-6 & 1-7] [see Box 1-1]

Facet Joints

Joints are interruptions in the skeleton where movement occurs; facet joints allow movement between the vertebrae. They are "synovial" type joints, as are most joints with detectable amounts of movement. Synovial joints are so-called because they are lined by a "synovial membrane" that produces fluid for lubrication and protection; a "joint capsule" surrounds and encloses the joint. Some synovial joints contain a "meniscus," a wedge-shaped crescent of solid tissue; one side of the meniscus attaches to the capsule and the free edge extends into the joint. [see Figure 1-8 C]

Box 1-1

---

(3) Structural reinforcement is provided by **ligaments**, tough and inelastic bands of tissue. The anterior and posterior "longitudinal ligaments" travel the length of the spine between vertebral bodies; with the shorter transverse ligaments, they tie adjacent vertebrae together. [see Figures 1-4 & 1-7]

(4) The primary function of **muscles** is not structural support or joining of bone to bone. Unlike ligaments, muscle tissue is elastic and, when stimulated by a nerve, contracts to pull two bony surfaces together. Muscles

Chapter 1

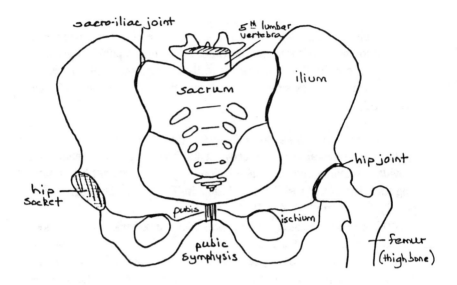

Figure 1-2. The pelvis and sacrum, front view.

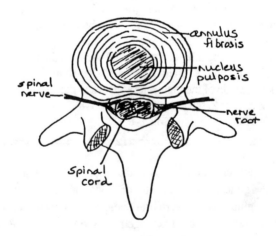

Figure 1-3. Vertebra with disk, spinal cord and nerve roots, top view.

16

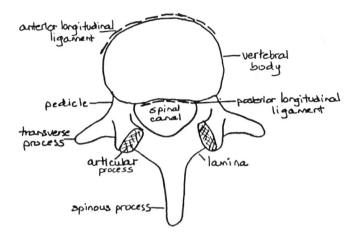

Figure 1-4. Vertebra with longitudinal ligaments, top view.

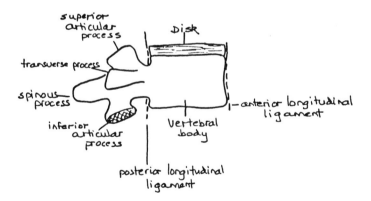

Figure 1-5. Vertebra with disk and longitudinal ligaments, side view.

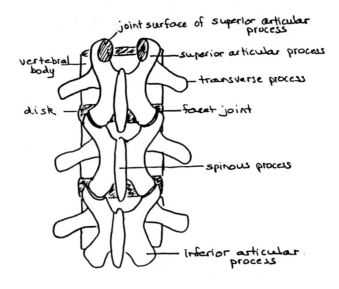

Figure 1-6. Section of the spinal column showing three vertebrae, back view.

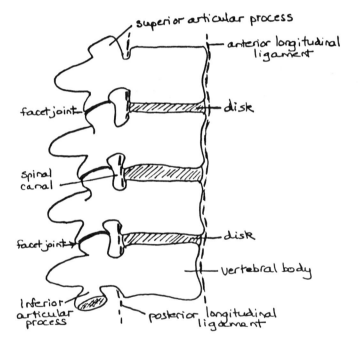

Figure 1-7. Section of the spinal column showing four vertebrae with disks and longitudinal ligaments, side view.

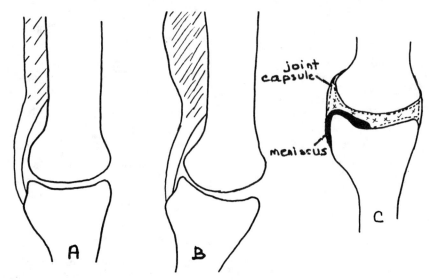

Figure 1-8. (A) Joint in extension with flexor muscle relaxed, side view. (B) Contraction and shortening of flexor muscle to move the joint into flexion. (C) Close-up side view of synovial joint with meniscus; dotted line represents synovial membrane and "x's" represent synovial fluid within the joint space.

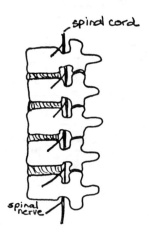

Figure 1-9. Section of the spinal column showing five vertebrae with disks, spinal cord and spinal nerves, side view.

provide strength for movement and postural holding. Some end in **tendons**, fibrous cords which attach muscle to bone. [see Figure 1-8 A & B]

(5) **Fascia** is connective tissue; it surrounds, permeates and joins all the structures and organs of the body. The brain and spinal cord are also covered by three fascia-type membranes, called "meninges". A liquid produced by the brain, "cerebrospinal fluid", fills the space between the two inner meninges to protect the brain and spinal cord.

Normal Movement of the Spine

"What a piece of work is man! . . . in form and moving how express and admirable!"
Shakespeare, *Hamlet*, Act 2, Scene 2

A passage called the **spinal canal** runs through the spinal column; within this spinal canal the **spinal cord** is located. The spinal cord consists of bundles of nerves which exit in pairs at each vertebra, carrying messages between the brain and body. [see Figures 1-3 & 1-9]

Sensation (including pain) travels from all parts of the body to the brain with information about the physical world. Specialized sensory nerves carry information about sight, taste, smell and sound. Nerve endings in the soft tissues of the body (the muscles, ligaments, and joint capsules) send the brain information about posture and movement. Feedback from these soft tissues plays a large role in both reflex and voluntary movement. These complex nervous system connections determine the response of the body's musculature to any stimulus, such as a shift in gravity, the decision to move or an injury.

Movement impulses travel in the opposite direction of sensation. Commands initiated in the brain travel down the spinal cord, out the nerve roots and along a nerve to the muscles, causing movement. When stimulated by a nerve impulse, muscles shorten and cause movement at joints by pulling two bony surfaces together. [see Figure 1-8 A & B] "Reflexes" are movements that happen so quickly they initially bypass the brain; a sensation travels inward only as far as the spinal cord, then immediately back to a muscle. For example, when someone touches a hot stove, her hand is jerked away before her brain can register pain.

Normal movement is limited by the shape, depth, type, and angle of joints, their ligamentous and muscular support and the presence of surrounding structures; due to all these factors different joints of the spine have different ranges of motion. The muscles that cross the small joints of the spine can cause movement in three planes.

- flexion/extension (bending and straightening)
- lateral flexion (bending away from the body's midline)
- rotation (twisting)

These facet joint movements are under voluntary control. Another kind of movement is called "joint play"; this refers to the small involuntary movements that occur within a joint in response to outside forces.

Normal Pain

"Pain is perception. Therefore all pain is in the brain." American Osteopathic Association[1]

Acute pain is a normal, protective response to alert the body to possible tissue damage. It is an unpleasant sensation, from discomfort to agony, caused by the stimulation of specialized nerve endings. Pain is primarily associated with physical injury, but since pain is a perception it may not be proportional or even directly related to an injury. The experience of hurting is a composite of physical, intellectual, emotional, motivational and situational reactions; factors other than tissue damage may directly affect the severity, tolerance and persistence of symptoms. In addition, pain does not necessarily correspond to the damaged area; it may move or change, and may or may not follow expected patterns of radiation. These are among the many reasons that pain may not be an accurate measure of the location and severity of an injury. They all need to be taken into consideration in the diagnosis and treatment of back pain.

Pain: An Unreliable Indicator of Pathology

1) Pain is highly subjective and influenced by emotional, intellectual and situational factors. A child may perceive the pain of a skinned knee differently in the presence of friends than in the company of his doting grandparents.

2) Accuracy of pain localization depends on nearness of the injury to the body surface. The pain from a rapped shin bone is well defined compared to the diffuse ache of an intestinal upset.

3) Pain perception does not necessarily correspond to the site of stimulation; pain can be referred to other structures. During a heart attack, severe pain may be felt down the left arm.

4) Different structures have different sensitivities to pain. [see Box 1-2]

Pain Sensitivity in Spinal Tissues

Some spinal structures are essentially without pain receptors or insensitive to pain; these include intervertebral disks, cartilage, vertebral bodies (unless invaded by cancer) and nerve roots. Pain responsive tissue (in the approximate order of sensitivity) includes the periosteum (outer covering of bone), joint capsules, synovial lining, ligaments (excepting the ligamentum flavum), subchondral bone (bone which lies beneath cartilage), tendons, nerves and nerve sheaths, fascia (connective tissue), cortical bone (bone which composes the outer layer of the shaft) and muscles.

In back dysfunction, the structures that usually give rise to pain are the anterior and posterior longitudinal ligaments, the outer covering of the nerve roots (the dura), the spinal muscles, the fascia of the muscles, the facet joints and the sacro-iliac joints.

Box 1-2

---

5) Severe pain in one structure can block pain from another structure. When someone stubs a toe, the pain from a headache is temporarily forgotten.

6) Pain is blocked by sensory stimulation. When an individual bangs her head, her tendency is to rub it. [see Box 1-3]

Gate Control Theory

Pain travels in small nerve fibers; it is usually blocked at the spinal cord by a steady volume of large fiber (sensory) impulses. When a strong enough painful stimulus occurs, the message of pain from the small pain fibers blocks the large fiber transmission to reach the brain and consciousness. Pain which would normally reach someone's awareness can in turn be blocked by increased levels of sensory stimulation. This view of pain perception is called gate control theory. It is the most common explanation for the pain relieving effects of acupuncture and TENS units.

Box 1-3

---

7) Pain can radiate, following nerve, muscle or embryological patterns of distribution.[2] "Sciatica" is felt as pain down the back of the leg, but it usually indicates a problem in the lumbo-sacral spine.

8) Painful structures can increase pain perception or can block pain in other structures from the same embryological segment. [see Box 1-4]

Embryological Pain Patterns

Pain patterns associated with deep injury may be related to the embryological development of the musculoskeletal system. When one structure is injured, other structures which originated in the fetus from the same mass of tissue are affected. The results may include an embryological pattern of increased muscle tone, hyperactive reflexes and increased skin sensitivity.[2]

Box 1-4

---

9) Pain perception can depend on the temporal or spatial summation of stimuli. An individual can comfortably perform many repetitions of a specific exercise and then suddenly feel pain the next time the motion is repeated.

10) Pain is inconsistent and may change in location and severity. The ache of an arthritic hip may wax and wane throughout the day for no apparent reason.

11) Pain is strongly influenced by the "placebo effect", the relief of symptoms caused only by the belief that one is receiving a pain-relieving treatment. The placebo effect may work through the production of "endorphins", or natural pain killers. [see Box 1-5]

Endorphins

Endorphins are opiate-like derivatives produced by the brain which have a pain-killing effect on the body. The following are thought to stimulate the body to secrete endorphins. . .

- tissue damage
- laughter
- exercise
- manual therapy
- the placebo effect

Box 1-5

---

12) Pain can persist after the organic cause has been treated and thought to be corrected. A whiplash injury may result in chronic pain despite the fact that no evidence of tissue damage remains.

Key Points - The Normal Back

The back is a complex unit made up of vertebrae, disks, facet joints, sacro-iliac joints, ligaments, muscles and connective tissue. Each structure assists in one or both of the dual functions of the spine – stability and movement. Back pain can be the result of dysfunction in any one of these structures; diagnosis and treatment require an understanding of their normal functions and interrelationships.

Pain is a normal protective mechanism of the body which signals potential tissue damage. However, pain is not a reliable guide to the location or extent of an injury. Identification of the primary site of pain can be difficult, even impossible. Every evaluation must be individualized.

Footnotes

1 American Osteopathic Association, informational literature
2 Stanley Paris, *The Spine*

Chapter 2 - Referrals From the Family Doctor

Medical Doctors

"It is not the business of the doctor to say that we must go to a watering place; it is his affair to say that certain results to health will follow if we do go to a watering place." Gilbert Keith Chesterton

MDs are required to complete four years of undergraduate education, four years of medical school, one year of internship, state licensure and continuing education credits – just to practice as GPs (General Practitioners). Most then add a two to seven-year residency and take national boards to become specialists. MDs have the whole of modern technology and science available to them for diagnosis and treatment; standard Western medicine is usually considered the only realistic option for preserving the lives of patients with certain diseases or injuries.[5]

A patient's family doctor, (usually a Family Practice or Internal Medicine specialist), may refer the patient to another physician with in depth training in a specific area. There are a variety of specialists who may be involved in the care of back pain patients.

Specializing Physicians

Neurosurgeons - referral for patients with clear signs of nerve or nerve root compression

Neurologists - referral with the presence of neurologic signs and symptoms other than those indicative of nerve root compression

Physiatrists (doctors of physical medicine) - referral for those with back pain related to non-surgical orthopedic or movement dysfunction

Rheumatologists - referral with signs of systemic rheumatoid disease or arthritis

Orthopedic surgeons - referral when x-rays show gross structural abnormalities or traumatic injury

Psychiatrists - referral when pain reports seem grossly exaggerated or abnormal, coping skills are inadequate or emotional factors are interfering with diagnosis and treatment

When radiographic and blood test studies are negative and there are no clear signs that make referral to a specialist appropriate, the patient probably falls into the "low back syndrome" category. This vague diagnosis is a frustration for both patient and doctor. In this case, the role of the primary care physician is to present the therapeutic options available and recommend a course of action, which the patient is free to accept or reject. As time passes, a review of the situation can lead to alternative recommendations. Doctor and patient work best as a team in the management of the patient's overall health needs.

Criticism of MDs

Physicians are often criticized for providing little help to patients with back pain. Complaints include the following:
- the expense and brevity of an office visit
- a diagnosis based only on x-rays
- a condescending attitude
- an approach that treats only the spine, ignoring the whole person
- an approach that treats only through the suppression of symptoms, ignoring the spiritual/emotional bases of pain

Illness does not merely affect the body; a person is influenced by culture, society, relationships, the perceived future, the roles one functions in, spiritual beliefs, intelligence and emotional makeup.[2] As Dr. Eric Cassel writes in the *The New England Journal of Medicine,*

"It is not possible to treat sickness as something that happens solely to the body without thereby risking damage to the person. An anachronistic division of the human condition into what is medical (having to do with the body) and what is nonmedical (the remainder) has given medicine too narrow a notion of its calling. Because of this division, physicians may, in concentrating on the cure of bodily disease, do things that cause the patient as a person to suffer."[2]

In the treatment of back pain, the family physician often lacks experience in approaches beyond conservative, symptomatic measures, (rest, heat, medications, etc.). What the family physician can do, however, is look for the diagnosable diseases that affect about 10-15 percent of back pain patients.[1,4] Practitioners who offer alternatives to standard Western medicine can miss the signs and symptoms that make referral to the appropriate medical consultant crucial. A physician is the best professional to find or rule out serious illness. A medical doctor can also offer the back pain patient an appropriate referral to a practitioner with the ability to provide individualized evaluation and treatment.

Therapies Through Physician Referral

"paindemons / skewer me / to the floor again / a quivering heap / lying in a quagmire / of tears and tangled hair; / face grotesque / with grimaces; / lips blue / around gritting teeth; / cursing, / fighting back, / doing the damned/ exercises- / i want my arm back!" Ardeana Hamlin, "Physical Therapy - First Sessions"

Physical Therapy
Physicians often refer back pain patients to Physical Therapy. PTs have a four-year Bachelor of Science or a graduate degree in Physical Therapy and take a state registry exam to become licensed. In some states PTs are now able to practice through direct access, without physician referral. Goals of PT are to. . .
- identify dysfunction (increased, decreased or abnormal movement)
- pinpoint affected structures
- relieve pain
- restore function, and
- prevent recurrence.

Although physical therapy is often equated with hot packs and whirlpools, these modalities are primarily used to prepare a patient for the more essential programs aimed at the restoration of normal movement.

PTs often specialize in the treatment of specific disabilities, but they are not certified as specialists. This means that a doctor's prescription is good for any registered therapist, but that therapists are not proficient in every therapeutic technique. The most effective PTs are those who have a well-rounded view of back pain and who don't become over committed to one philosophy.[6] In addition to treating the specific dysfunction, PTs also need to look at the overall status of the patient and address posture, body mechanics, physical conditioning, etc.

Patients with back pain all used to be treated with the same regime, ("Williams flexion exercises"), but it is now widely recognized that each program needs to be individualized. Although PTs do not diagnose disease, they should be proficient at diagnosing dysfunction. A physical therapist who is familiar with the range of approaches for "low back syndrome", (Williams versus McKenzie exercise programs, mobilization techniques, identification of Sacro-Iliac Joint Dysfunction, etc.), has the best chance of localizing a patient's problem and providing successful treatment.

Occupational Therapy

The educational requirements for occupational therapists are similar to those of PTs – a four year B.S. or graduate degree with state registration and continuing education credits. Occupational therapy has traditionally not played as large a role as physical therapy in the treatment of back pain, but this is changing. OTs have expertise in a large variety of developmental and rehabilitative services; they are part of the team at pain clinics and involved in the return to work of patients injured on the job. OTs may provide therapy for pain coping, pain management, the psychological complications of pain, work hardening, evaluation of functional capacity and adaptation of the home or work environment.

Kinesiotherapy

Kinesiotherapists work under the auspices of a physiatrist, (a doctor of physical and rehabilitative medicine). They are commonly employed in the Veteran's Administration system, but also work in the private sector. KTs have a bachelor's degree and 1,000 hours of clinical training; they take a national certification exam and participate in continuing education. Areas of expertise include physical fitness training, exercise, disabled driver training and acute and chronic patient care.[3] In VA hospitals where there is a shortage of physical therapists, KTs have been accused of performing treatments beyond the scope of their training. Gait training, therapeutic exercise and evaluation of strength and range of motion are treatments more appropriately carried out by a PT.[7]

Key Points - Referrals from the Family Doctor

The family doctor is often the first person a back pain patient sees. MDs tend to recommend conservative treatment; they often do not have expertise in other forms of therapy. Family doctors may refer patients to specializing physicians or to physical therapy for treatment. They can rule out potentially serious illness and can help patients coordinate an overall health care program.

Footnotes

1 *The Back Letter*, Vol. 4, No. 3
2 Eric Cassell, "The Nature of Suffering and the Goals of Medicine"
3 Terry Dimick, "Kinesiotherapist Responds"
4 Richard DonTigny, "Function and Pathomechanics of the Sacroiliac Joint"
5 Mills & Finando, *Alternatives in Healing*
6 David Reese, "Keep PT the Art That It Is"
7 Ellen Strickland, "Trouble with KTs"

Chapter 3 - Doctors Who Manipulate the Spine

Osteopaths

"The DO has an advantage over the MD in that the DO is trained in manipulative therapy." Bob Jones[12]
"During the last decade, osteopathic schools have de-emphasized manipulation." Randolph Kessler, PT and Darlene Hertling, PT[14]

Osteopathy differs from general medicine in its emphasis on the role of the musculoskeletal system in health and disease and in its use of spinal manipulation. Osteopaths also take a holistic approach to medicine, focusing on the patient as a whole, versus a specific illness. Educational requirements include three years at the college level, a four-year degree program, one year of internship, state licensure and continuing education; 45 percent of osteopaths go on for specialization.[1] DOs can now prescribe drugs, do surgery and provide a whole range of medical services. In fact, DOs and MDs have come to work more and more closely together; many osteopaths practice medicine in almost identical fashion to MDs and refer patients to specializing physicians and therapists. Manipulation, the distinctive feature and the original basis of the profession, is currently being de-emphasized in osteopathic schools. [see Box 3-1]

> ## The Basis of Osteopathy
> In 1874 Andrew Still founded Osteopathy, a medical approach based on the premise that "body structure governs function and disturbances of structure lead to disturbances of function". [22] The musculoskeletal system, in addition to providing framework and support, has a major influence on the body's ability to maintain wellness. When this structure is healthy, the circulatory and nervous systems carry maintenance and repair capabilities to the rest of the body; the body is then able to be self-regulating and self-healing in the face of disease. Improper muscle functioning can impede blood and nerve supply, causing illness in other parts of the body. Manipulation of the musculoskeletal components can return the whole body to health through its effects on the circulatory and nervous systems. Some osteopaths recommend regular manipulation as a preventative measure for greater well-being and lowered susceptibility to illness in general. [12]
> ### Box 3-1

Osteopathic Diagnosis: Somatic Dysfunction

While more and more DOs now work as specialists in a hospital setting, there are still many osteopaths whose practice consists primarily of treatment through manipulation. They believe that close to 95 percent of back pain is caused by what they call "somatic dysfunctions". [23] These are functional, or non-structural, disorders of the musculoskeletal system; they are associated with pain, muscle spasm, structural malalignment and impaired mobility. Because unwellness is reflected throughout the body, illness or injury of any structure or system can cause somatic dysfunction. Once present, somatic dysfunctions deplete energy, lower resistance and can produce problems in the internal organs. In other words, a somatic dysfunction may. . .

1) trigger disease in the rest of the body

2) perpetuate disease by interfering with recovery

3) indicate the presence of internal disease, or

4) once initiated, can itself become a secondary disease, remaining even after the precipitating factor is gone.

Somatic dysfunction can only be diagnosed through palpation (hands-on examination) of musculoskeletal structures and the careful observation of movement. Although evaluation and manipulative treatment focus on the muscles, the final effects occur within the nervous system, affecting the whole body. Manipulation restores function through relaxation and lengthening of muscles; this then decreases the abnormal sensory input to the nervous system. The body is then able to regain a normal, balanced state so that unwell parts of the body can repair themselves. Chronic pain or illness results when somatic dysfunction is not properly diagnosed and treated.[23]

A recent study of patients receiving osteopathic manipulation produced the following results. The treatment significantly benefitted some patients whose pain had lasted two to four weeks, but did not benefit those with shorter or longer episodes of pain. In addition, after four weeks of treatment no advantage could be detected for those patients who had received osteopathic manipulation compared to patients who received no manipulation.[3] Manipulation as a treatment for back pain is controversial; its rationale, benefits and risks are discussed later in this chapter.

Chiropractors

"Vertebral subluxations [asymmetries] *are found in every sick, malfunctioning body."* John Langone[17]

"Asymmetry of the human body is not the exception, but the rule." James McGavin, PT[19]

Chiropractic and osteopathy are often confused; both emphasize the importance of the musculoskeletal system in overall health, both developed in the late 1800s, both have names that are not self-explanatory and both use manipulation to treat disease.[12] Chiropractors, however, are not licensed to provide a full range of medical services; they are limited to diagnosis and treatment of structural changes in the spinal column. The concern of the profession is the relationship between impaired movement of vertebrae and the nervous system, and its effect on health.[5] Chiropractic has both vehement advocates and critics; it is considered by medical and osteopathic physicians to fall considerably short of comprehensive medicine. Some consider this an asset and view chiropractic as a profession which offers patients safer or less toxic alternatives to prescription medications and surgery. [see Box 3-2]

The Basis of Chiropractic

Founded by Daniel Palmer in 1895, chiropractic is based on the "Law of the Nerve"; this states that the body has all the necessary components for health and that disease occurs when nerve impulses are reduced or changed. Misaligned spinal bones interfere with the normal pattern of nerve impulses, decreasing the body's efficiency and resistance to infection. Loss of alignment of the vertebral column can result from such factors as gravitational stress, strains, postural or movement asymmetry, developmental defects or nervous system irritations. Since spinal malalignments interfere with nerve and blood supply to the rest of the body, these off-centerings of the vertebrae can then cause disease. Once produced they become the focus of sustained pathology. For this reason, chiropractors treat all human ailments through manipulation of the spine.[20]

Box 3-2

Chiropractic Diagnosis: Vertebral Subluxation

A "subluxation" is the name for an off-centering or malalignment of one vertebra relative to other vertebrae. Subluxations are functional defects - they may not show on a standard x-ray but are apparent through movement limitations. Unlike osteopaths, chiropractors palpate for vertebral displacement rather than decreased mobility. To further pinpoint subluxations, chiropractors take full body x-rays in the positions in which the patient's pain is present; x-rays of the relaxed body in the lying down position are not useful because at rest the effects of muscle contraction and gravity are eliminated and subluxations are least in evidence. In addition to x-rays and palpation, chiropractors may use a "thermograph", a diagnostic technique which measures spinal heat. A subluxation interferes with blood supply, causing a drop in temperature; cold spots may also result from nerve compression, muscle spasm or areas of tenderness. Thermographs also identify hot spots resulting from inflamed nerves and muscles.

Variation Among Chiropractors

All chiropractors agree that subluxation plays a role in disease, but there are two schools of chiropractic thought. "Straights" stick to the "Law of the

Nerve" and treat all disease with manipulation; assessment is based solely on subluxations so they see no need to diagnose disease.[5] "Mixers" tend to be more liberal, treating other joints, using other treatment forms and making more modest claims. Mixers are more apt to accept the limitations of manipulation and supplement it with a variety of modalities - heat, cold, water, electricity, vitamin therapy, mechanical devices, diet, exercise, massage, psychotherapy, acupuncture or any combination of these.

Today, the straight chiropractic faction is said by some to be hurting the profession; it is seen as irresponsible to claim to provide primary health care and yet see no need to diagnose. There are only two colleges of straight chiropractic in the U.S. and these are not recognized by the accrediting agency for chiropractic schools.[5] The chiropractic profession seems to be moving away from its original rigid philosophy. Many chiropractors no longer claim to treat all diseases through spinal adjustments. Subluxations are more broadly defined to be - neurological or circulatory involvement due to (1) structural displacement of vertebrae **or** (2) abnormal function (movement) in a spinal segment. The mechanisms involved are recognized to often go beyond a simple pinching of a nerve by a displaced vertebra.[5]

Opposition to Chiropractic

Much criticism is leveled at chiropractic, and it focuses on a variety of concerns.

1) **Education.** Past standards for education were dreadful - in 1942 one could still purchase a chiropractic degree through the mail. Admission requirements were low, teachers and science courses inferior, and a 1972 study concluded that "deficiencies were too pervasive to permit an adequate educational experience".[6] Chiropractic education has improved since then; requirements now call for two years of college and four years of professional school. Diagnosis is now in the curriculum, but without hospital training or residency, chiropractic students (and instructors) don't see the range of diseases that DOs and MDs do. This means that the ability to diagnose contraindications to treatment is still a weak area; "straights" don't diagnose at all.[5] There is also minimal training in pharmacology; this is relevant[*] because many chiropractors prescribe vitamins and discourage the use of drug therapy.[6]

2) **Radiation.** 90 percent of chiropractic patients are x-rayed, (compared with 3 percent who see MDs).[6] Chiropractors are looking for structural

malalignment to treat. However, slight postural shifts in standing can cause asymmetry during filming, giving the appearance of a minor subluxation. In addition, asymmetry exists in normal, pain-free spines. Chiropractors often take x-rays in full side-bending; people normally don't function in this extreme range, so these x-rays don't represent the spine in its typical position.[21] Some feel the massive radiation used by chiropractors is unwarranted and is used primarily to impress patients.[6]

3) **Philosophy.** Using manipulation to treat all diseases through its effects on the nervous system is the original philosophy of chiropractic; such effects are inconsistent and inconclusive when subjected to clinical trials.[22] The only parts of the nervous system accessible to manipulation are the 26 pairs of spinal nerves. This leaves 12 pairs of cranial nerves, 5 pairs of sacral nerves, the spinal cord, brain and parasympathetic nervous system which cannot be affected by manipulative treatment. Furthermore, there is no scientific evidence that minor subluxations impinge on spinal nerves. Even some advocates of chiropractic now state, *"No responsible chiropractor today claims to cure organic disease through adjustments of the spine."*[5]

4) **Risk.** Doctors should weigh risks against benefits before initiating treatments with possible side-effects. When chiropractors use manipulation as a universal therapy, this is not a consideration, and a patient may be harmed by inappropriate treatment. Four percent of patients in one study suffered direct injuries from chiropractic, from increased pain to serious nerve damage.[6] There is even a slight risk of stroke associated with cervical adjustments.[5] Chiropractic is also blamed for keeping patients from appropriate, timely medical treatment in cases of serious illness.

There is no question that chiropractors help some back pain patients, but the reasons are highly controversial. Many people visit their chiropractors regularly, claiming significant relief from minor back pain and stiffness. Others go regularly for general health maintenance. One author states, *"Preventive treatment for children is important, and regular check-ups are recommended."*[20]

Consumer Reports, an organization whose purpose is impartial testing of products and services, has studied the chiropractic profession. Its editors have written that chiropractic is a significant hazard to many patients and recommends the following for those who pursue the approach:[6]

1) Limit it to appropriate muscular complaints.

2) Refuse x-rays and vitamin therapy.

3) By-pass chiropractic altogether for the treatment of children.

4) Avoid chiropractors who make claims about miraculous cures, who never make referrals to other health practitioners and who use scare tactics about what may happen if treatment is delayed.

Osteopathic and Chiropractic Manipulation

"Manipulation can provide dramatic relief of pain, spasm and restriction of motion." Paul Kaplan, MD & Ellen Tanner, PT[13]

"Many patients do report dramatic relief, others recover despite manipulation." Charles Fager, MD[10]

Manipulation is used by both osteopaths and chiropractors to treat patients with back pain. However, not only do their manipulative techniques differ, but their philosophies as well. Osteopaths manipulate to correct a dysfunctional state of muscles and chiropractors to restore normal bony alignment. Because their views on the cause of back pain differ, so do their treatment methods. [see Box 3-3]

Manipulative Techniques

Osteopaths manipulate by localizing their force at the level of impaired mobility; thrust is applied with the minimum force necessary, usually in the direction of limitation. If the limitation is too great, more gentle techniques are used. The patient is positioned so that the joints on either side of the hypomobile segment are locked through ligament tension or facet joint position. A thrust is then imparted to restore mobility to that segment.[7,22]

Chiropractors palpate for vertebral displacement rather than decreased mobility. They apply pressure to the bone itself, using force to shift the vertebra back into place.[7] Unlike the protective locking used by osteopaths, pressure is applied to vertebral bony processes in order to open the space between the vertebrae; a high velocity thrust is then delivered to realign the segment.[22]

Box 3-3

Chapter 3

A popping or cracking sound often accompanies manipulation. This may be caused by the breaking of adhesions. Another cause is a pressure change when joint surfaces are suddenly forced apart. A carbon dioxide gas bubble, liberated from the synovial fluid inside the joint space, collapses with a crack.[15,22]

Criticism of Manipulation

Chiropractic and osteopathic manipulation can produce dramatic, positive results for some back pain patients. Both professions have their own explanation for the successful effects of treatment - correction of malalignment or of a somatic dysfunction, respectively. Other back experts theorize that manipulation is useful for some conditions and is a valid approach, but that its success is instead due to:

- restoration of joint play
- displacement of a disk fragment
- stretching of a tight muscle
- tearing of soft tissue adhesions, or
- relief of muscle spasm.

There is no definitive proof that any of these are correct.[6]

Manipulation's scientific rationale is unconvincing to many.[8] Critics of manipulation feel that any positive results produced have one of the following alternative explanations.

1) The doctor-patient relationship. There is psychological value in the laying on of hands and the offer of a sympathetic ear in a non-hurried atmosphere, (unlike that found in many medical offices). Patients who have been unable to receive a firm diagnosis elsewhere are reassured to put themselves into the hands of someone who is confident about the cause of the pain and the appropriate treatment. The placebo effect depends on inspiring this confidence.

2) Most illness is self-limiting regardless of what treatment is applied.

3) Manipulation blocks pain perception in two ways. The sensory stimulation produced by manipulative techniques inhibits the transmission of pain impulses to the brain. The nerves carrying pain sensation are blocked at the spinal cord by faster sensory impulses. In addition, manipulation is thought to stimulate the production of endorphins, the body's own painkillers. Both of these forms of pain relief are only temporary.

A number of practitioners feel that high velocity thrust is inappropriate for most spinal conditions and that most patients do better with mobilization.

40

[see Box 3-4] These experts recommend that manipulation not be used at the beginning of treatment and never with a very painful joint or a joint being protected by muscle spasm. It may be appropriate for certain patients to later progress from mobilizations to manipulations.[18] A general rule for practitioners who use manipulation/mobilization is to use the gentlest technique which will produce the desired results.[18]

Mobilization
Mobilization is performed within a patient's available range of motion and is of lower speed and amplitude than manipulation. Mobilization techniques involve graded, gentle, rhythmic movements at specific joints, done within the patient's tolerance. The joint is passively taken to the limit of its available range where a series of gentle stretches or progressive reciprocal movements are performed to gradually relieve restriction.[22]
Box 3-4

There should be an immediate change in mobility or pain level with manipulation; if relief is not obtained within about three treatments, manipulation will probably not be effective.[2,4,11] An increasingly widely held view is that manipulation has positive short-term effects for some, especially when combined with other treatments, but that long-term benefits are questionable.[6,9,16] In other words, manipulation may speed improvement but doesn't affect the long-term prognosis for many back patients.

Key Points - Doctors Who Manipulate the Spine

Back pain patients are often confused about which type of doctor to consult. Medical doctors, osteopaths and chiropractors all have advocates and critics. The education that MDs and DOs receive is now very similar and includes years of hospital training. Chiropractic evaluation and treatment is limited to structural changes in the spinal column. Both chiropractors and osteopaths emphasize the role of the musculoskeletal system in health and disease, and both treat back pain with manipulation. Osteopaths manipulate to correct somatic dysfunctions and chiropractors to correct vertebral subluxations. Included in this chapter are the concerns frequently expressed concerning the safety and effectiveness of manipulation.

Footnotes

1   American Osteopathic Association, informational literature
2   "Approaches to Musculoskeletal Problems: Focus on the Low Back" Symposium, Donald Fraser
3   *The Back Letter*, Vol. 4, No. 9
4   Rene Cailliet, *Low Back Pain Syndrome*
5   David Chapman-Smith, "Chiropractic - A Referenced Source of Modern Concepts, New Evidence"
6   Consumer Reports Books, *Health Quackery*
7   James Cyriax, *Textbook of Orthopaedic Medicine*
8   Richard Deyo, "Conservative Therapy for Low Back Pain"
9   Richard DiFabio, "Clinical Assessment of Manipulation and Mobilization of the Lumbar Spine"
10 Charles Fager, "Beware the Quick Fix for Back Pain"
11 David Imrie, *Goodbye Back Ache*
12 Bob Jones, *The Difference a D.O. Makes*
13 Kaplan & Tanner, *Musculoskeletal Pain and Disability*
14 Kessler & Hertling, *Management of Common Musculoskeletal Disorders*
15 W.H. Kirkaldy-Willis, *Managing Low Back Pain*
16 Klein & Sobel, *Backache Relief*
17 John Langone, *Chiropractors: A Consumer's Guide*
18 G.D. Maitland, *Vertebral Manipulation*
19 James McGavin, "The McKenzie Approach to Spinal Pain"
20 Mills & Finando, *Alternatives in Healing*
21 Stanley Paris, "Physical Signs of Instability"
22 Stanley Paris, *The Spine*
23 William Wyatt, DO, literature for patients

Chapter 4 - Comparing Health Care Providers

"Fashions in therapy may have some justifications; fashions in diagnosis have none."
Robert Herrick

Comparing the Doctors

"Illness is the most heeded of doctors: to goodness and wisdom we only make promises; pain we obey." Marcel Proust

Some medical doctors, osteopaths and chiropractors have a tendency to look down on the other two professions, each believing their own approach to be the most enlightened. Their relative successes in eliminating back pain, as rated by the Klein and Sobel survey of back pain patients, are equally unimpressive.[6]

percentage providing dramatic long-term help
- family doctors - 8 percent
- osteopaths   - 7 percent
- chiropractors (manipulation only) - 5 percent
                              (total care) - 14 percent

percentage ineffective or making patient feel worse
- family doctors - 66 percent
- osteopaths   - 57 percent
- chiropractors (manipulation only) - 44 percent
                                        (total care) - 44 percent

Physiatrists (MDs specializing in physical and rehabilitation medicine) have more success than any of these doctors, with 33 percent providing dramatic long-term relief and only 14 percent ineffective or making the patient feel worse. Physical therapists also score higher with ratings of 34 percent and 27 percent, respectively. Physiatrists treat patients with a broad range of back conditions. They use physical modalities and exercise in addressing movement problems and work closely with physical therapy. Unfortunately, physiatrists are few in number, practicing mostly in large cities.[6]

For patients with negative x-rays and blood tests, a common frustration with medical doctors is their unwillingness to provide a concrete diagnosis. Negative diagnostic tests may be interpreted as meaning that nothing serious is wrong. The patient may be asked about stress, causing him to fear that the doctor thinks the pain "is all in my head". Osteopaths and chiropractors, on the other hand, know exactly what's wrong, (somatic dysfunction and subluxation, respectively), and how to treat it, (manipulation). Finding a practitioner who can confidently pinpoint the problem comes as a great relief - unless the treatment is ineffective. Unfortunately, manipulation alone seldom provides long-term relief.[2,4,6]

It is important to remember that pain relief is only one goal when seeking medical help; diagnosis is the other. The people whose back pain indicates serious illness can eventually be firmly diagnosed through laboratory or radiographic tests and are likely to receive effective treatment for their conditions. Other back patients may not get pain-relieving therapy from their physicians, but may receive significant help in other areas. Their physicians can rule out disease, make referrals for effective treatment, offer emotional support and assist in the development of a plan for pain management.

The common denominator for success among the three types of doctors seems to be the following:[6]

1) an ability and willingness to explore the situations that increase pain and relate symptoms to specific spinal structures

2) the application of appropriate, individualized treatment based on the

results of the evaluation

3) consideration of the patient's daily living habits and general health, with recommendations concerning posture, body mechanics, exercise, etc.

or

4) making a referral to a practitioner who has these skills.

Traditional Versus Alternative Medical Approaches

"Care more for the individual patient than for the special features of the disease." Sir William Osler

The treatments for back pain are many and their classification is not always clear. The approaches which are most commonly and traditionally used to treat people with back problems can very generally be said to target the back versus promoting overall health. These methods also tend to fall into the realm of standard Western medicine and to be administered by registered health professionals.

There is much talk about alternative ways to treat health problems; usually what is meant is alternatives to surgery and prescription medications. It is frequently stated that Western medicine treats only symptoms, ignoring their causes, or treats only diseases, ignoring the patient. Many alternative approaches are "holistic"; they emphasize that the physical, mental, emotional and spiritual sides of a person must all be addressed in treatment. Every person is considered to be an integral part of the creative force of nature and the universe; health involves an increasing awareness of that universal energy.[5]

"Everything is one; there are no accidents. Labeling anything as a chance happening resulting from either randomness, coincidence or luck merely exposes our ignorance of the interrelationships that brought it about."[3]

Holistic practitioners place great emphasis on removing the obstacles, (physical, psychological or spiritual), that prevent the body from healing itself. Patients are responsible for their own health and disease;[5] with the support and guidance of the health practitioner, they are helped to make the changes in their lives that will promote recovery. Other concepts common to many alternative and holistic approaches include the uninterrupted flow of energy through the body, balance among the various influences on the body, and the role of the body's connective tissue in dysfunction.

These less traditional treatments are becoming more popular; they are administered by a variety of practitioners, many who are licensed professionals and some who are self-proclaimed and unregulated. Alternative healers do help some back pain patients; the ones who best serve the whole person are able to accept the following concepts:

1) Standard Western medicine is not merely the pharmacological or surgical repression of symptoms.

2) Patients should not be led to expect miracles from alternative approaches, then held responsible if the treatment is unsuccessful.

3) Every patient and every health problem is different; a single treatment approach is unable to help every patient.

4) Every person has a right to his or her own spiritual philosophy; holistic professionals who provide physical treatment should beware of tying spiritual/world view counseling to clinical techniques.[1,5]

The medical profession is often unwilling to take alternative approaches seriously. On the other hand, many holistic practitioners condemn traditional medicine as uncaring, ineffective or harmful. A rigid or defensive attitude on the part of any health practitioner is unfortunate. It is in a patient's best interest to feel comfortable exploring a variety of approaches to determine which will be most effective. Some people will be helped by conventional approaches and some by alternatives, and probably many by a combination. Whatever treatment can relieve a patient's pain and dysfunction, be it visualization or back exercises, should be supported by the practitioner, be he Rolfer or neurologist.

Key Points - Comparing Health Care Providers

It is recommended that to rule out potentially serious conditions, patients with back pain consult physicians with access to the full range of diagnostic services. Survey results indicate that all three types of doctors are unsuccessful in providing long-term, dramatic help for most back pain patients. Success is highest for those professionals who can individualize diagnosis and treatment and address the patient's overall health needs.

Traditional and alternative approaches to the treatment of back pain are many and varied. Health care providers are often unwilling to objectively consider therapies outside their own area of expertise; many are defensive about perceived criticism and unable to admit their limitations. Individualization of diagnosis and treatment means that practitioners put the patient's welfare ahead of a rigid philosophy of health care.

Footnotes

1   Benanti & Ellis, "Holistic Medicine a 'Crisis' for PTs"
2   Rene Cailliet, *Low Back Pain Syndrome*
3   Annemarie Colbin, *Food and Healing*
4   Richard DiFabio, "Clinical Assessment of Manipulation and Mobilization of the Lumbar Spine"
5   Nina Kim, "Holistic Medicine Requires Different World View"
6   Klein & Sobel, *Backache Relief*

Chapter 5 - Diagnostic Evaluation

Radiographic Tests

"Back about a couple of months ago, I had a little touch of lumbago,
So I called on my doc to see what he'd suggest.
And he said, 'Man, it's plain to see the hospital's the place you oughta be,
Cause what you need is good old fashioned rest!'" Doug Harrell, "Hospitality Blues"

A diagnosis is reached by combining a patient's history and physical exam with radiographic and laboratory studies. There are a large variety of diagnostic procedures available to the physician; several are commonly used when a patient complains of back pain. These are most helpful for ruling out serious medical conditions or for confirming what is already suspected from the history and physical exam. However, for the "low back syndrome" patient, results of diagnostic testing are often negative or falsely positive and are of limited value.[4]

X-Rays

As discussed in Chapter 3, chiropractors routinely use full spine x-rays for diagnosing vertebral subluxation. MDs use x-rays to screen for conditions such as cancer, TB, osteoporosis and fractures, but once such diseases are ruled out, x-rays tell a doctor very little.[5] They do not provide information about disks or other soft tissues. Often back pain is explained by the anomalies or arthritic changes revealed on x-ray, but such findings occur with equal frequency among people without symptoms. As both patient and doctor are anxious to find an explanation for the patient's pain, it is understandable that both accept a diagnosis based only on x-rays. However, numerous studies have revealed the poor correlation, in both lumbar and cervical areas, between x-ray abnormalities and pain or dysfunction.[9] By the fifth decade, 90 percent of men and 60 percent of women show x-ray evidence of degenerative changes;[9] these are usually not responsible for a sudden onset of back trouble.[7] Some experts now say that x-rays are not necessary unless an episode of acute back pain lasts beyond 6-7 weeks.[2]

Other Non-Invasive Radiographic Tests

MRI (Magnetic Resonance Imaging) uses magnetic fields and radio waves to examine soft tissues; unlike x-rays which only visualize bones, MRI can image soft tissue in any plane with clear contrast. MRI is an expensive, relatively new technique with no known side-effects.

CAT Scans (Computerized Axial Tomography) are multiple x-rays combined by a computer into one picture; they show a cross-section of both soft tissue and bone. Forty percent of people over 40 have abnormal CAT scans. 35 to 45 percent of CAT scans are false positive for back pain pathology, including 20 percent which show ruptured disks in people who have never had back pain.[1,2]

Thermography is a controversial technique which identifies cold spots or hot spots around the spine; it hinges on the assumption that nerve root irritation produces changes in skin temperature. Although it is used by some practitioners, including chiropractors, its reliability is unproven.[1,4]

The advantage of CAT scans and MRI is in determining the size and location of a ruptured disk, or for patients with extensive arthritis, stenosis (narrow spinal canal), tumors, infections, etc. CAT scans are particularly useful for identifying lateral nerve root compression from . . .

- bone spurs (see Chapter 10, "Spondylosis")
- lateral disk ruptures (see Chapter 7, "Prolapsed and Ruptured Disks")
- entrapment between an enlarged subluxed facet joint and the back of the vertebral body[8] (see Chapter 8, "Facet Joint Dysfunction").

However, CAT scans and MRI are performed extensively, often without satisfactory indication. When these tests show simple bulging of disks, they may be used as indications for surgery; this has led to many unnecessary operations.[4] Bulging disks are common in people with and without back pain and may have nothing to do with a patient's symptoms. Doctors can learn as much with a history, physical exam and possibly x-rays, reserving these expensive procedures for patients with strong evidence of nerve or nerve root compression.

Myelograms

The myelogram was the major diagnostic technique used to detect nerve root compression before CAT scans and MRIs became available. It has the disadvantage of being invasive, painful and having possible side-effects. In a myelogram, cerebrospinal fluid is withdrawn from the space which surrounds the spinal cord; dye is then injected and an x-ray taken to identify possible nerve root or spinal cord compression by disk, tumor, bone spur or stenosis. [see Figure 5-1] Some people with no history of backache or neck pain have evidence of defects; myelography has an accuracy rate of 70-85 percent.[6] It is generally reserved for pre-operative testing.

Other Invasive Radiographic Tests

CAT-Myelograms are tests in which dye is injected as in a myelogram and the patient then receives a CAT scan. One indication for this test is when lateral nerve root compression is suspected.

Other procedures also involve dye injection into different structures for diagnostic purposes.

Diskography - Dye is injected into a disk; if the dye leaks out it indicates that the disk is ruptured. Diskography is less effective than other techniques for identifying a herniated disk, but may be the best tool for finding herniations associated with disk degeneration.[1]

Chapter 5

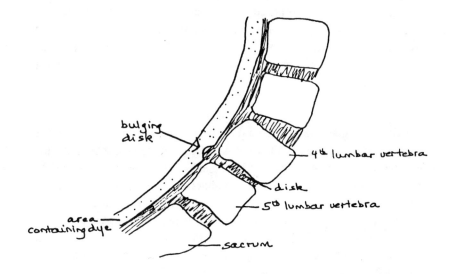

Figure 5-1. Representation of a myelogram showing a prolapsed disk between the 4th and 5th lumbar vertebrae which may or may not be causing pain.

52

Epiduralgram - The area outside the outermost covering of the spinal cord, the dura, is injected; with a ruptured disk, a bulge shows up on x-ray.

Epiduralvenogram - The vein in the groin is injected; this test assumes that with a nerve root compression the vein as well as the nerves will be affected. This procedure causes less discomfort than injection in the spinal region.

Anesthetic Injection - Injection of dye can be combined with an anesthetic agent to show which site, when injected and numbed, will result in the elimination of pain. This is done to localize the pain-causing structure.

Bone Scans involve injection of a radionuclide dye into a vein; bone scans are rarely positive if x-rays are negative, but are effective for identifying bone tumors and infections.

EMG (Electromyography) shows involuntary electric waves generated in muscle fibers and recorded by a needle electrode inserted into the muscle. Different nervous system diseases have distinctive EMGs. Nerve root compression causes specific electric patterns ("fibrillation potentials") in affected muscles, but some feel EMG is seldom reliable in defining the compression's location.

The Physical Examination

"When he finally got off of that talkin' jag, he pulled out a little black doctor's bag
And gave me the darnedest physical I ever had.
He beat on me with a hammer and tickled my feet and did some things I better not repeat
And 'bout the time he finished another boy in white walked in." Doug Harrell, "Hospitality Blues"

Because of the limited value of radiographic testing for people with low back syndrome, the physical exam is of major importance; too often it tends to be superficial.[3] Patients are often stereotyped into three groups - those with neurologic signs have a disk rupture, those without have a muscle strain and those with abnormal x-rays have arthritis; unfortunately it's not that clear-cut.

The recommended procedure to follow in a thorough physical exam is the following.[3]

1) Know the normal structure and movement of the spine.

Chapter 5

2) Recognize deviations from normal.

3) Establish the exact mechanisms that initiate the pain.

4) Be able to reproduce the pain by reproducing these mechanisms.

By identifying pain-causing movements or positions and understanding how they relate to the anatomy and function of the spine, the cause of back pain can be clarified. The where, when and how of the pain (position, action, motion, time of day, stress, fatigue, state of mind, etc.) are all factors to be considered in diagnosis.

The following may all be part of a thorough physical exam for the patient with unremitting back pain.

1) **Pain**
- patient's description and visual representation of the pain (pain drawing)
- patient's report of what aggravates and relieves symptoms
- mechanisms that reproduce these symptoms on examination
- description of pain patterns and direction of radiation
- areas of tenderness and pain referral patterns on examination
- comparison of pain on flexion versus extension
- comparison of pain on left versus right trunk movements
- effects of movement of spinal and peripheral joints on pain
- effects of repeated movements on pain
- effects of straight leg raise (this test is discussed in Chapter 7, "Prolapsed and Ruptured Disks").

2) **Movement**
- patient's ability to move while undressing
- patient's willingness and ability to move during examination
- asymmetry or abnormality of gait
- asymmetry or abnormality of trunk and peripheral joint movements
- muscle strength (including calf muscles)
- patient's ability to walk on heels and on tiptoe
- comparison of active versus passive movements of spine and hips

3) **Structure**
- passive range of motion of spine, hips and straight leg raises
- presence of instability or hypermobility in spinal joints
- patient's spinal configuration and posture
- body build and muscular development
- presence of muscle spasm, muscle atrophy or abnormal muscle tone
- peripheral joint abnormalities (including flat feet)
- leg length difference
- differences in thigh or calf circumferences
- structural deformities, including pelvic obliquity

4) **Neurologic Signs**
- reflex testing (including ankle jerk)
- abnormal sensations (including big toe and lateral foot)
- referral pattern of abnormal sensations
- rectal sphincter tone and perirectal sensation
- patient's report of abnormal sensations

5) **General Health**
- medications being taken
- strength of peripheral pulses
- extent of patient's discomfort
- prostate or pelvic examination (noting vaginal discharge, tenderness or masses)
- examination for abdominal or renal tenderness
- evaluation of heart, lungs and general health

One goal of a physical examination is to establish a formal diagnosis; for people with back pain it has another function. The specific findings of the physical exam can determine the appropriate treatment. Treating a "diagnosis" with a routine approach may help some patients while aggravating others; patients react differently to the same disease and treatment must be individualized. This is especially true if the patient's only diagnosis is "low back syndrome". There are many treatment approaches for back pain; the results of the physical exam can determine which of these can best address the specific structural limitations or movement dysfunctions which have been identified.

Key Points - Diagnostic Evaluation

X-rays are too often used as the primary method of determining the cause of a patient's back pain. Diagnosis may be based on abnormalities or degenerative changes if they are present; these findings were probably present before the onset of pain and occur in many pain-free people. X-rays can only identify bony pathology; when the spine is normal on x-ray, doctors and patients may assume there is no physical problem. Myelograms, CAT scans and MRI can visualize bulging or ruptured disks, but these procedures should generally be delayed until a patient is clearly a surgical candidate. They are most helpful for confirming what is already suspected from the history and physical exam. Patients with low back syndrome who hope to get a definitive diagnosis for their back problems through diagnostic testing are frequently disappointed.

Due to the difficulty in pinpointing the cause of back pain, patients may be undiagnosed or misdiagnosed. A thorough physical exam is the most important way to determine not only the cause of back pain, but also the appropriate treatment. The exam should identify specific pain-causing movements and positions and relate them to the anatomy and function of spinal structures. Treatment based on these findings has the best chance of obtaining successful results.

Footnotes

1 *The Back Letter*, Vol. 4, No. 5
2 "Approaches to Musculoskeletal Problems" Symposium, Robert Boyd
3 Rene Cailliet, *Low Back Pain Syndrome*
4 Charles Fager, "The Neurosurgical Management of Lumbar Spine Disease"
5 David Imrie, *Goodbye Back Ache*
6 Bernard Jacobs, "Low Back Pain: The Orthopedist's View"
7 Kaplan & Tanner, *Musculoskeletal Pain and Disability*
8 Kirkaldy-Willis & Hill, "A More Precise Diagnosis for Low Back Pain"
9 John Rice, et al., "Low Back Pain: The Rheumatologist's View"

Chapter 6 - Differential Diagnosis

"Then he asked me a million questions or more 'bout every kind of sickness I'd had before,
But every question that I asked him he just ignored.
Aunt Susie had the dropsy, but I'll never know what the devil that's got to do with lumbago,
And the questions about my private life made me mad." Doug Harrell, "Hospitality Blues"

Ruling Out the Diagnosable Diseases

Back pain is a symptom present in a wide variety of health problems. Before assuming that a patient is one of the estimated 85-90 percent[1] who falls into the "low back syndrome" category, a physician may need to consider and rule out any number of the following conditions or diseases. These can be differentiated from the low back syndromes because most can eventually be definitively diagnosed through radiographic, laboratory or other tests. With a verifiable diagnosis, the recommended treatment approach is much less controversial. A discussion of these conditions is beyond the scope of this book; they are listed here to emphasize how complicated the differential diagnosis of back pain patients can be. [see Box 6-1]

Conditions Causing Back Pain

Trauma - spondylolysis (defect in the spinal arch of a vertebra), spondylolisthesis (the same defect on both sides with anterior slipping of the vertebral body), fracture of coccyx, vertebral body or transverse process, lower sacral nerve root compression* (symptoms include sexual dysfunction and intense leg pain)

Inflammation - ankylosing spondylitis or Marie Strumpell's (especially in young men complaining of persistent pain around the sacroiliac joint), rheumatoid arthritis, gout, fibrositis,** lupus (SLE), Reiter's Disease, psoriatic arthritis, enteropathic arthropathies (colitis, Crohn's Disease)

Metabolic Disease - osteoporosis (thin bones), osteomalacia (soft bones), pathological fractures, diabetic neuropathy

Degenerative Disease - hip disease, Schmorl's node (fragment of disk protruded into vertebral body), osteoarthritis, myelopathy (central nervous system changes), hyperostosis (bone spurs), temporal-mandibular joint disease (TMJ)

Congenital Disorders - facet tropism (asymmetry), sacrolization of fifth lumbar vertebra (elongated transverse process forming a false joint with the sacrum), lumbarization of first sacral vertebra, leg length difference, stenosis (narrow spinal canal), untreated scoliosis (lateral curvature of the spine), spina bifida (unjoined vertebral arch)

Circulatory Problems - aortic aneurysm, vascular insufficiency (e.g., from stenosis), varicose veins, peripheral vascular disease, arteriosclerosis

Infections - disk space infections, pyogenic disease, epidural abcess, TB, chronic osteomyelitis, fungal infections, heavy metal poisoning, Lyme disease, arachnoiditis (possibly secondary to injection of contrast dye for myelography)

Tumors - benign (neurinoma, meningioma, neurofibroma, neurilemmoma, cord tumors), malignant (multiple myeloma, osteoid osteoma, metastases, neural tumors)

Referred Pain - genitourinary tract conditions (VD, urinary tract infections, prostate disease, tipped uterus, uterine fibroids, endometriosis, pelvic tumors and infections), inflammatory or obstructive conditions of abdomen (involving kidneys, pancreas,

(continued)

---

lymph nodes, GI tract, liver, bladder), sclerosis, cancers, viral pneumonia, heart or lung disease

Psychoneurotic Problems - pain memory, pain behavior, hysteria, malingering, depression, "profound sensitivity syndrome" (allergic reaction to body's own hormones causing emotional over-reaction)

*Lower sacral nerve root compression is briefly discussed in Chapter 7, "Prolapsed and Ruptured Disks"

**Fibrositis is briefly discussed in Chapter 9, "Strains, Sprains and Spasms"

Box 6-1

Low Back Syndrome

Once the diagnosable diseases have been ruled out, patients are usually left with a diagnosis of low back syndrome, or one of the conditions which fit into this category. These syndromes involve pathology of the following spinal structures.

1) Intervertebral Disks - Commonly called slipped disks, this condition results when the inner part of the disk pushes through the outer fibers. If this causes a bulging, it is called a **prolapsed disk**; if a fragment pushes all the way through, it is a **ruptured disk**. Ruptured disks may or may not cause nerve root compression.

2) Facet Joints - The moveable joints linking the vertebrae are the facets. They are subject to a variety of **facet joint dysfunction** such as sprain, inflammation, arthritis and instability. One of these joints may also become displaced and jammed; when this happens the soft tissues of the joint can be pinched. This is called acute locked back syndrome.

3) Soft Tissue - The non-structural parts of the spine include muscles, tendons, ligaments and fascia. Injuries to muscles or ligaments are called **strains** and **sprains**, respectively. When a muscle stays tightened to protect itself or other structures, it is in **spasm**. The fascia, or connective tissue of the body, is now thought by some practitioners to be important in causing or perpetuating pain and dysfunction.

4) The Whole Spine - Degenerative disk disease, arthritis and degenera-

tive disease of the spine are all terms used to describe the changes of aging; these affect vertebrae, disks, facet joints and soft tissues. The combination of these degenerative changes is called **spondylosis.**

5) Sacro-Iliac Joints - The SI joint has limited movement, but it can become wedged and irritated, especially if it is excessively mobile to begin with. This syndrome is called **sacro-iliac joint dysfunction.**

6) Piriformis Muscle - This condition also involves soft tissue, but is localized to a specific muscle. If the piriformis muscle goes into spasm, it can compress the sciatic nerve, causing both localized and referred pain. This describes the **piriformis syndrome.**

There are many who think years of poor posture has the most dramatic impact on causing any of these six syndromes and is the chief culprit in most low back and neck problems. Poor posture is known to predispose disks, muscles and joints to injury and to speed the degenerative process of the spine.

The many structures of the spine are interrelated and injury to one can initiate pain and dysfunction in the others. Experts on back pain disagree widely on which is usually the site of the primary pathology. With six specific syndromes to choose from, one would expect that identifying the problem would be routine. The following factors complicate the issue.

1) Different distinct syndromes can yield the same symptoms.

2) Syndromes producing characteristic symptoms may occasionally present in an atypical way.

3) When facet joints are involved, the disk is affected and vice versa.

4) Muscle spasm may accompany spinal pain no matter what the cause.

5) Degenerative changes on x-rays may be unrelated to pain.

6) Radiating pain does not necessarily imply nerve root compression.

7) Pathology in one structure can cause mechanical problems in any weight-bearing joint.

8) Piriformis muscle spasm can cause sacro-iliac strain and vice versa.

9) Irritated tissue in a sclerotome (deep tissues innervated by the same spinal nerve) can cause irritation in all tissues of that sclerotome.

10) Sclerotomes and dermatomes (skin area innervated by the same spinal nerve) do not correspond exactly.

Due to individual differences and the interrelatedness of spinal structures, pinpointing the site of primary pathology may be impossible. However, specific symptoms are usually associated with specific spinal structures; for many patients careful evaluation can lead to a definitive diagnosis. The following guidelines for differential diagnosis are very general and not meant to present a complete picture of the low back syndromes; exceptions are not uncommon. [see Box 6-2]

Differential Diagnosis - Low Back Syndrome

Onset of Pain
- Sudden - facet joint dysfunction, muscle spasm, SIJD (sacroiliac joint dysfunction)
- Gradual - spondylosis, soft tissue strain, piriformis syndrome
- Sudden or gradual - disk prolapse or rupture (disk rupture here assumes nerve root compression)

Type of Pain
- Dull, achy - soft tissue strain, spondylosis, SIJD, piriformis syn.
- Sharp, grabbing - facet joint dys., muscle spasm
- Dull and sharp - disk prolapse (aching into leg), disk rupture (sharp down leg); either type of pain in low back area

Location of Pain
- Diffuse - soft tissue strain, muscle spasm
- Localized - disk prolapse or rupture (precise down leg), facet joint dys. (tender over facet), spondylosis (aching of lumbosacral spine and hips), SIJD (dull pain over SI joint, buttock and posterior thigh), piriformis syn. (tender over piriformis muscle and sciatic nerve distribution)

Radiating Pain
- Radiating pain dominant - disk rupture
- Lack of radiation - soft tissue strain, muscle spasm, spondylosis, facet joint dys.
- Radiating pain less significant than localized pain - disk prolapse, SIJD, piriformis syndrome

(continued)

Pain Aggravation
- worse after rest (stiff) - soft tissue strain, muscle spasm, spondylosis
- worse with trunk flexion - disk prolapse and rupture
- worse with extension - facet joint dys., spondylosis
- worse with repetitive motions - SIJD, piriformis syn.

Neurologic Signs
- Presence of neurologic signs - disk rupture
- No neurologic signs - all other syndromes

Straight Leg Raise Test
- Positive SLR and crossed SLR - disk prolapse and rupture
- Negative SLR - facet joint dys., soft tissue strain, muscle spasm, spondylosis
- Other - SIJD (contralateral SLR), piriformis syndrome (SLR becoming positive with forceful hip internal rotation)

Symmetry/Asymmetry of Symptoms
- Bilateral - spondylosis
- Unilateral - disk prolapse and rupture
- Bilateral or unilateral - facet joint dys., soft tissue strain or spasm, SIJD, piriformis syn.
- Asymmetric pelvic landmarks - SIJD
- Scoliosis - disk prolapse and rupture, facet joint dys.

Pain referred from non-spinal tissue differs from the low back syndromes in that it is persistent, unrelieved by rest and unassociated with activity; it does not follow a pattern of distribution typical of that associated with spinal structures.

Box 6-2

The patient's response to treatment procedures may also help determine a diagnosis. For example, the effect of manipulation on pain can be dramatic with facet joint and sacroiliac dysfunction; the response to injection of an anesthetic agent is effective in pinpointing facet or piriformis syndromes. Usually, passive extension exercises relieve disk pain, heat eases muscle spasm, etc. A patient may or may not come through the diagnostic process with a firm diagnosis, an explanation for the pain or the site of the pain pinpointed. The more accurate the understanding of the symptoms, the easier it is to select the appropriate treatment approach.

PART 2 concerns the "low back syndromes", their cause, pathology, symptoms, diagnostic rationale and treatments. These syndromes involve the structures of the low back, but most of what is said about disks, facet joints, muscles and degenerative changes of the spine apply to neck pain as well. An understanding of these conditions is important in helping patients judge the appropriateness and effectiveness of treatment.

Key Points - Differential Diagnostic

There are many, many conditions which may cause back pain, but in only about 10-15 percent of patients does this symptom lead to a definitive diagnosis through radiographic, laboratory or other tests. The remaining back pain patients are left with a diagnosis of "low back syndrome" or one of the six conditions which fit into that category. Interrelationships of spinal structures, similarity of symptoms among syndromes and atypical combinations of symptoms make identification of the primary site of pain difficult. Guidelines for differential diagnosis between the low back syndromes are presented, but these are only generalizations; every patient is different and every evaluation must be individualized. Patients who understand the meaning and rationale of their diagnoses are the best equipped to judge the appropriateness and effectiveness of treatment.

Footnote

1   Richard DonTigny, "Function and Pathomechanics of the Sacroiliac Joint"

PART 2 - THE LOW BACK SYNDROMES

Chapter 7 - Prolapsed and Ruptured Disks

Rene Cailliet, MD, 1962 - *"In the treatment of disk disease . . ., the first exercise is the movement of knee to chest. After each leg separately is flexed to the chest, the action of both knees to chest is added."* [4]

Rene Cailliet, MD, 1988 - *"It becomes obvious that flexion exercises can intensify (disk protrusion). The exercises that are of value in disk protrusion are those of lumbosacral extension and avoidance of flexion type exercises."* [5]

Intervertebral disks sit between the bodies of the vertebrae and provide cushioning and shock absorption for the spine; they have a tough fibrous outer ring (the **annulus** fibrosis) and a soft gelatin-like center (the **nucleus** pulposis). [see Figure 7-1] There is no such thing as the infamous "slipped" disk; disks do not slip out of place - only the nucleus moves. Injury occurs when the nucleus is forced through torn annular fibers. When the annulus bulges out from the pressure of the nucleus it is called a prolapse or protrusion. When the annular fibers tear completely, nuclear material exits

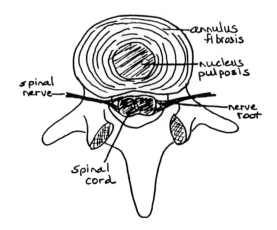

Figure 7-1. Vertebra with disk, spinal cord and nerve roots, top view.

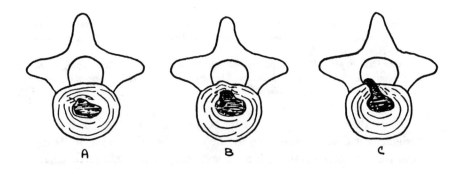

Figure 7-2. Increasingly severe levels of disk dysfunction, top view. (A) Tearing of inner annular fibers. (B) Tearing of inner and outer annular fibers with bulging of annulus into spinal canal. (C) Rupture of annular fibers with extrusion of nuclear material into the spinal canal.

into the spinal canal; this is called a rupture, herniation or extrusion. [see Figures 7-2 & 7-3] With a rupture, nuclear fragments may or may not press on a nerve root. [see Figure 7-4] Trauma can also cause the nucleus to herniate up or down into the vertebral body of an adjacent vertebra, but this is uncommon.

The typical disk injury occurs when an individual is bending forward and twisting. Disk problems may also build up gradually as a result of excessive sitting, common in modern society.[9] The flexed position pushes the nucleus posteriorly, stressing the annular fibers; over time this sets the stage for an acute injury. Symptoms are caused by pressure against pain sensitive structures, specifically the outer annular fibers, the posterior longitudinal ligament and the coverings of the nerve root (the dura). [see Figures 7-3 & 7-4] It has also been theorized that pain may result from a leakage of nuclear material which inflames the nerve root chemically, even without direct compression.[5]

Disk injuries are categorized by the direction and extent of nuclear protrusion and its effects on surrounding structures. There are at least five levels of disk derangement. [see Figure 7-2]

1) inner annular tear - The nucleus extrudes only through the inside ring of annular fibers, bulging against the pain sensitive outer annular fibers.

2) outer annular tear - The nucleus extrudes into the outer annular fibers.

3) outer annular protrusion (posterior or posterolateral) - The annulus bulges out, pressing on the posterior longitudinal ligament and possibly the dura (the covering of the nerve root).

4) annular tear with nuclear extrusion (posterior or posterolateral) - Nuclear material exits through tears in the annulus with pressure on the posterior longitudinal ligament and possibly the dura.

5) nerve root compression - Nuclear material presses on the dura and nerve root causing pain and neurologic signs in the arm or leg, (numbness, weakness, decreased reflexes).

Common Symptoms of a Disk Prolapse or Rupture
- pain developing immediately or shortly after injury, sometimes building up gradually to become apparent upon rising the next morning
- pain increased by sneezing, bending, coughing and straining
- pain usually on one side only
- pain worse in sitting and flexion (bending)

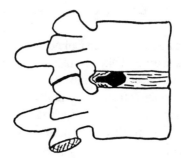

Figure 7-3. Section of vertebral column showing 2 vertebrae with a prolapsed disk bulging into the spinal canal and compressing the posterior longitudinal ligament, side view.

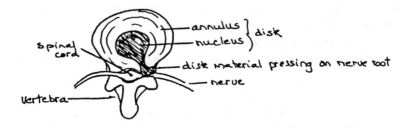

Figure 7-4. Vertebra, top view, with a ruptured disk compressing a nerve root.

- pain relieved by rest
- flexion markedly restricted
- severe, protective muscle spasm contributing to a loss of the normal lumbar lordosis
- presence of a lateral spinal curve, usually away from the involved side

Common Symptoms of a Disk Prolapse
- deep, aching, poorly localized pain from pressure on annular fibers and the posterior longitudinal ligament
- straight leg raise test positive due to the position of flexion stressing the disk [see Box 7-1]
- referral of pain to back and groin versus along the distribution of the sciatic nerve
- aching into the leg

Common Symptoms of a Disk Rupture
- sharp, radiating and well-defined pain down the back of the leg ("sciatica"*) which follows the path of the sciatic nerve
- neurologic signs (numbness, weakness, decreased reflexes) which follow a pattern of spinal nerve distribution
- straight leg raise test positive from increased pressure on the nerve root [see Box 7-1]
- crossed straight leg raise test positive due to entrapment of the nerve root [see Box 7-1]

*Sciatica alone is not considered a neurologic sign or proof of a true rupture; sciatica may be present with other spinal pathology.

Straight Leg Raising

The straight leg raise (SLR) is a test done to diagnose disk rupture. The patient is put into a position of hip flexion with knee extension; a positive SLR is said to occur if pain is elicited or increases. SLR is positive with a disk prolapse because the flexed position increases the posterior movement of the nucleus. The position itself can also produce pain with other kinds of pathology.

A true SLR also incorporates ankle dorsiflexion (foot toward face) and neck flexion in the test position; this is the most significant neurologic test for disk rupture. If these additional components cause radiating pain it means that the dura (covering of the nerve root) is being stretched; this positive dural sign indicates disk rupture with nerve root compression. A positive "crossed SLR" elicits radiating pain on the opposite leg; this is caused by a significant entrapment of the nerve root by a ruptured fragment which prohibits the lateral movement normally produced by the test position.

Box 7-1

A patient may feel better if a protrusion progresses to a true rupture because there is suddenly less pressure on the pain sensitive annulus and posterior longitudinal ligament. However, with a rupture, nerve root compression, neurologic signs and sciatica can develop. This is a more serious problem; it has the potential for nerve root injury with permanent effects. Because of this possibility, pain cannot be the major diagnostic factor or even concern when a rupture is suspected.

People over age 60 rarely have ruptures of the nucleus; by the fifth decade the water content of the nucleus decreases and cracks begin to form in the annulus. Disk ruptures still occur, but from tears and prolapses of the annular fibers.

Sacral Nerve Root Compression

Because the sacral vertebrae are fused into one bone, the sacrum, there are no sacral disks or ruptures. However, lower sacral nerve root compression can occur; it can be caused by a fall, accident or pregnancy. It reportedly involves the following symptoms.[2]

- pelvic pain
- vaginal discharge
- impotence
- buttock pain and "paresthesias" (abnormal sensations)
- radiating pain in one leg and paresthesias in the other, or pain and paresthesias in both legs
- bladder problems
- inability to have orgasm

Patients usually focus on the sharp leg pain, neglecting to mention the less intense symptoms which follow the sacral nerve root (S-2) pattern. For this reason the injury may be mistaken for a ruptured disk.[2]

Box 7-2

Treatment for Prolapsed and Ruptured Disks

Bedrest - Total bedrest is not essential for disk protrusion, but avoidance of excessive activity is advisable. Initially, if virtually all motion is impossible, a period of bedrest in a relatively extended position with minimal weight-bearing may be necessary. The patient may feel comfortable in the fetal position at first because the annulus is drawn taut, moving the bulge away from the nerve root. This position, however, increases pressure on the nucleus, so the patient should avoid excessive flexion. Even with a rupture, one week of total bedrest is considered the maximum.[1] As soon as possible, periods of rest should be interspersed with short periods of standing and walking.

Manipulation - Manipulation, though performed regularly for disk disorders by osteopaths and chiropractors, is controversial. Gentle, nonrotary mobilization techniques are thought safe, but many recommend against using more vigorous approaches.[8] Manipulation is especially risky when it causes

71

worsening neurologic signs.

Exercise - "Williams flexion exercises" used to be routinely recommended as the treatment for all types of low back pain, but it is now generally agreed that flexion exercises should be avoided with disk problems. Flexion exercises can increase the posterior bulging of the nucleus and further tear the annulus.

Extension, on the other hand, forces the nucleus centrally, away from the nerve roots. In general, gentle repetitive stretch and compression through exercise speeds healing of annular fibers. However, if the disk has ruptured, extension may cause increased pain due to further compression on the fragment; in this case exercises are contraindicated. [see Box 7-3]

Exercise Program for Disk Prolapse

(If extension does not reduce pain, this program is contraindicated.)

- avoidance of flexion and rotation in the acute phase, including sitting
- "press-ups," or passive hyperextension exercises, in the acute phase (The back extensor muscles are not used to perform this exercise; the patient presses up from the prone position using the arms.) [see Figure 7-5]
- with a posterolateral nuclear protrusion, incorporation of a lateral shift with extension, in order to move the nucleus centrally
- learning correct sitting posture and use of a lumbar roll
- gentle flexion prefaced by extension after 5-7 days*

This exercise routine, when applied to the right patients, boasts a 97 percent improvement rate.[9]

*The disks absorb more water during sleep, so that flexion exercises done in the morning can result in 300 percent more stress on the lumbar disks than the same movements later in the day.[3]

Box 7-3

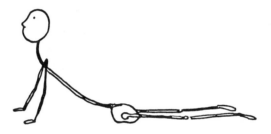

Figure 7-5. A "press-up"; passive hyperextension of the spine performed to relieve a prolapsed disk.

Injection - Patients with nerve root compression can receive a steroid injection into the space surrounding the spinal cord and nerve roots. This treatment is called an epidural injection. It decreases pain without significantly interfering with sensory or motor nerves. Advocates of epidural injections claim it provides immediate pain relief in 80 percent of patients;[10] the effects gradually dissolve over the following six months. One study, however, found no difference in pain relief between patients receiving an epidural injection and those who were injected with a placebo.[6] One risk of epidural injection is incorrect placement of the needle, which happens up to 25 percent of the time.[10] Serious complications include infections or inflammation of the meninges (the three outer coverings of the brain and spinal cord).[6]

Surgery - Surgery is a common treatment for ruptured disks, but too many operations are performed due to misinterpreted radiographic findings.[7] Radiographic testing should not be the basis of a diagnosis, but merely confirm the clinical picture. Bulges seen on CAT scans and MRI often result in unnecessary disk removal; even with myelography there are false positives and negatives. Only 1 percent of back pain patients have an actual ruptured disk.[5]

The only findings which call for referral of a back pain patient to a surgeon are the presence of unremitting radiating pain to the limbs and the presence of neurologic signs (numbness, weakness and decreased reflexes). Conservative treatment is recommended for at least four weeks before surgery is seriously considered. The decision to operate demands: (1) clear, objective clinical evidence of nerve root compression; (2) confirmatory radiographic tests; (3) a failure to respond to conservative therapy; and (4) an appropriate psychological profile. Immediately following surgery, the patient should receive full passive straight leg raises every two hours to avoid nerve root adhesions which can interfere with recovery.[9]

Cauda Equina Syndrome

The one area in which conservative treatment is contraindicated is the "cauda equina syndrome" in which there is compression on sacral nerves. A massive extrusion in this area can result in bladder symptoms; in this case relieving the compression is urgent. A "neurogenic bladder" involves loss of bladder emptying tone, of bladder capacity sensation and of sphincter function. Unless this condition is treated promptly, (some say within hours), permanent, irreparable bladder dysfunction can result. For this reason, perianal sensation and rectal tone should be a part of every physical examination when disk rupture is suspected.[5]

Some experts credit disk deterioration or injury as being the most common cause of persistent back pain. They believe that even vague back symptoms are often due to minor disk injury, with insufficient nuclear protrusion to be diagnosed. Such problems may then become increasingly serious due to neglect in the early stages. Whether or not it is the primary cause of back pain, disk dysfunction has a dramatic influence on all the structures of the spine.

Key Points - Prolapsed and Ruptured Disks

A disk is prolapsed when its soft gelatin-like center, the nucleus, pushes into its surrounding outer fibers, the annulus. A rupture occurs when the nucleus pushes completely through torn annular fibers into the spinal canal; here it may press on a nerve root, causing radiating symptoms to the leg. The flexed position aggravates disk problems. The recommended treatment to correct the bulging of the nucleus is extension exercises. Bedrest, manipulation and surgery are other treatment approaches for ruptured or prolapsed disks, but their use is more limited and not appropriate for all disk patients.

Footnotes

1   "Approaches to Musculoskeletal Problems: Focus on the Low Back" Symposium, Jane Derebery
2   *The Back Letter*, Vol. 4, No. 4
3   *The Back Letter*, Vol. 4, No. 8
4   Rene Cailliet, *Low Back Pain Syndrome*, 1962 ed.
5   Rene Cailliet, *Low Back Pain Syndrome*, 1988 ed.
6   John Cuckler, et al., "The Use of Epidural Steroids in the Treatment of Lumbar Radicular Pain"
7   Charles Fager, "The Neurosurgical Management of Lumbar Spine Disease"
8   G.D. Maitland, *Vertebral Manipulation*
9   James McGavin, "The McKenzie Approach to Spinal Pain"
10 Arthur White, "Injection Techniques for the Diagnosis and Treatment of Low Back Pain"

Chapter 8 - Facet Joint Dysfunction

"The facet joint is the principle seat of initial spinal pathology. This author has long been convinced that the facet joint is the most common source of low backache and sciatica." Stanley Paris, PT[4]

"It is unlikely that the symptoms of most low back pain could be due to lesions of the facet joints." James Cyriax, MD[1]

Facet joints link the bones of the spinal column together; four articular processes of one vertebra form joints with two superior articular processes of the vertebra below it and two inferior articular processes of the vertebra above it. [see Figures 8-1 and 8-2] These are "synovial" joints, lined by a synovial membrane that produces fluid for lubrication and protection; a capsule surrounds and encloses the joint. Some synovial joints contain a meniscus, a wedge-shaped crescent of cartilage and fibrous tissue; one side attaches to the joint capsule and the free edge extends into the joint. [see Figure 8-3] Synovial joints exists for the purpose of movement between

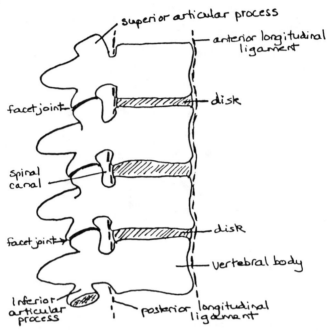

Figure 8-1. Section of the spinal column showing four vertebrae with disks and longitudinal ligaments, side view.

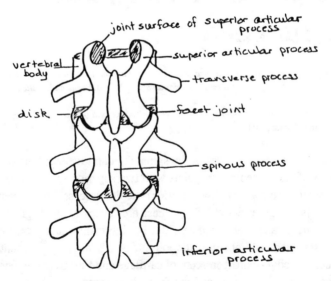

Figure 8-2. Section of the spinal column showing three vertebrae, back view.

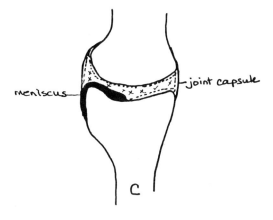

Figure 8-3. Close-up side view of synovial joint with meniscus; dotted line represents synovial membrane and "x's" represent synovial fluid within the joint space.

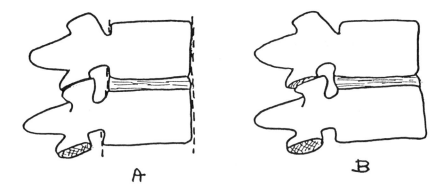

Figure 8-4. (A) Section of the spinal column showing two vertebrae, side view. (B) Subluxation of the facet joint causing narrowing of the spinal canal, with possible pinching of the soft tissues of the joint or entrapment of a spinal nerve against the vertebral body or disk.

bones; the shape and depth of the joints are two factors which determine the amount and type of movement. Facet joints can slide, compress together or pull apart, depending on the movement of the trunk.
- flexion - Facets on both sides slide and the joint surfaces separate.
- extension - The joints are jammed together.
- rotation - The facet on the side to which the person is rotating separates and the opposite side is compressed.

Facet joints are subject to the same problems as other synovial joints.

1) **Sprain** - A sprain usually results from a traumatic injury in which supporting ligaments are torn or stretched. Treatment involves an initial period of rest alternated with pain free movement; this allows time for healing to occur and prevents adhesions from developing.

2) **Inflammation** - Inflammation often follows a sprain or occurs with chronic postural strain; these stresses cause swelling of the joint. As with strain, the joint needs time to heal with rest and gentle movements.

3) **Degenerative Disease** - Arthritic changes in the joint can occur with aging. The causes and treatment of degenerative disease of the joints of the spine is discussed in Chapter 10, "Spondylosis."

4) **Hypermobility** - Abnormally excessive movement of joints can result from poor posture, congenital defects, severe trauma or by overtreatment with manipulation or stretching. It is also found in segments next to a hypomobile (less mobile than normal) segment. Symptoms of hypermobility include pain when attempting to hold a weight-bearing posture, pain relief upon moving out of a static posture, and a localized angulation or catch during forward bending instead of smooth trunk movement.[3] The treatment for hypermobility includes mechanical support, postural and strengthening exercises, and avoidance of stressful motions (such as rotation) at the unstable segment.

5) **Hypomobility** - Abnormally limited movement of joints can result from poor posture, spinal malalignment or an injury which elicits protective muscle spasm. Hypomobility also occurs when there is a subluxation or displacement of opposing facet joint surfaces; the result is jamming or locking of the joint. [See Figure 8-4] In the process, the meniscus, synovial membrane or joint capsule may become nipped. This is sometimes called "acute locked back syndrome"; other names are facet impingement or block. It occurs suddenly with intense pain in the low back which makes straightening up difficult.

Symptoms of Acute Locked Back Syndrome
- sudden onset
- sharp twinge or catch
- pain either unilateral (on one side) or bilateral (on both sides)
- tenderness over facet and in lower lumbar area
- pain worse in standing and with extension
- pain relieved in flexion
- absence of neurologic signs or radiating pain
- negative straight leg raise test
- minimal leg discomfort
- loss of normal lumbar curve (lordosis)
- lateral flexion toward involved side

Since facet joints jam in extension and open in flexion, the flexed position relieves pain while extension aggravates it. This fact is very helpful in distinguishing facet dysfunction from a prolapsed disk where pain is usually relieved by extension and increased by flexion.

Nerve Entrapment in the Lateral Recess

This syndrome occurs when a spinal nerve is entrapped between an enlarged subluxed superior articular process and the back of the vertebral body and disk. [see Figure 8-4] It involves the nerves between either the L 4-5 or the L 5-S 1 vertebral segments, and produces buttock and leg pain. Where manipulation is helpful in diagnosing other facet subluxation, it is not in patients with a lateral recess entrapment; the CAT scan is the best diagnostic tool to use.[2]

Box 8-1

The proponents of facet pathology as the major cause of back pain believe that facet injury produces subsequent changes in the whole spine. When one spinal joint is affected, movement in adjacent joints is altered, causing stress on other structures. Muscular, ligamentous and disk pathology are thought to often be secondary to earlier facet dysfunction.[4] Facet joint pathology can have a variety of effects.
- protective muscle spasm, restricting motion
- the development of adhesions, restricting motion

- entrapment of the meniscus between the facets which can alter its shape, permanently restricting motion
- decreased nutrition to the disk from restricted motion
- increased sheering forces on adjacent disks from restricted motion in one spinal segment
- disk degeneration from decreased disk nutrition and increased sheering forces

Some experts are skeptical that back pain could be due to facet dysfunction and doubt that two parallel surfaces can lock. They reason that if patients did have facet joint dysfunction. . .
- spinal deviation from muscle spasm would not be away from the painful side
- pain would not be central
- pain would not increase with cough, neck flexion or straight leg raise as the facet doesn't interfere with the nerve root
- pain would not occur with flexion or lateral flexion to the painless side as this gaps the joint
- there would not be neurological deficits.

Eliminating all the patients who do have the above symptoms, opponents of facets as primary sites of back pain believe that only one in 100 patients could have facet pathology.[1]

Treatment of Facet Joint Hypomobility

Facet joint hypomobility or acute locked back syndrome is a condition usually treated with manual therapy, i.e., mobilization or manipulation. The goal of treatment is to (1) realign opposing joint surfaces, or (2) restore "joint play," the small involuntary movements within a joint. A loss of joint play can result due to tightness or adhesions of soft tissues which surround a joint, (joint capsule, connective tissue or ligament). In cases where tissue is pinched between the joint surfaces, a maneuver in flexion is used to separate the joint and free the trapped structure.

Manipulation and mobilization have strong proponents, strong opponents and a wide range of techniques to choose from. Manual therapy's rationales, applications and pros and cons are discussed in Chapter 3, "Doctors Who Manipulate the Spine".

Key Points - Facet Joint Dysfunction

The facets are the moving joints of the spinal column. They are subject to the same problems as the other synovial joints of the body. A common affliction is hypomobility, a decrease in the normal amount of movement. One cause is a subluxation or jamming of the joint, which may cause soft tissue to be pinched. There is controversy over whether or not this "locked back syndrome" occurs and its frequency of occurrence. The usual treatment for a hypomobile facet joint is manipulation or mobilization.

Footnotes

1   James Cyriax, *Textbook of Orthopaedic Medicine*
2   W.H. Kirkaldy-Willis, "A More Precise Diagnosis for Low Back Pain"
3   Stanley Paris, "Physical Signs of Instability"
4   Stanley Paris, *The Spine*

Chapter 9 - Strains, Sprains and Spasms

"To help make your spine strong and stable you have muscles." David Imrie, MD[9]

"Rather than being dependent on strong muscles, a strong spine has strong ligaments and stable facet joints." Glenna Batson, PT[2]

Even among those who agree that muscles play the major role in back pain, the specific mechanism involved is controversial. Muscle induced back pain may be due to . . .

1) traumatic muscle strain

"The most common low back syndrome, often associated with trauma with no radiological abnormalities, is ascribed to (spinal) muscle spasm." [7]

2) weak muscles from poor physical conditioning

3) tension

4) chronic muscle fatigue from poor posture and body mechanics

"80 percent of low back pain is caused by muscles that are weak, tense, fatigued or all three." [15]

5) tight muscles from poor physical conditioning

"Decreased flexibility affects spinal stability, making the occurrence of sprain, strain or spasm more likely." [1]

6) obesity

"Flaccid, distended abdominals from being overweight increase stress on the spine by 50 percent." [1]

7) spasm secondary to pathology of other spinal structures.

Probably it is impossible to make such fine distinctions, and the role of the musculature in back pain involves a combination of the above factors - acute strain and tension superimposed on poor posture, poor physical conditioning and degenerative changes. Two additional muscle-related syndromes are thought by some practitioners to be responsible for back pain; these are even more controversial.

8) tightening and thickening of the fascial sheath which surrounds muscles [see Box 9-1]

Fascial Restrictions and Back Pain

Fascia, the largest and most pervasive organ system of the human body, exists below the skin, around and infused with all structures and organs. In response to an orthopedic injury, the fascia shortens and thickens; it is likewise affected by stress. If stress-related postures and movement patterns persist, extra fascia will be built up and will hold these dysfunctional positions.[16] The fascial restrictions then perpetuate the pain and abnormal movement patterns, even if the original cause is resolved.

Box 9-1

---

9) trigger points (tender fibrous bands located in muscles) characteristic of the syndrome called "fibrositis" [see Box 9-2]

Fibrosis

Fibrositis, (also called myofascial pain syndrome, fibromyalgia or fibromyositis), is a response to various underlying clinical conditions. It involves pain and stiffness in muscles, joint areas, bony processes and connective tissue. The tender fibrous bands found in muscle tissue are called trigger points. Inflammation or abnormal lab findings are not present. Fibrositis is also characterized by chronic sleep disturbance; this may indicate a physiologic alteration in the brain's pain mechanisms. Some experts have associated fibrositis with a type A personality, or with various orthopedic abnormalities.[17,18]

Box 9-2

Whether muscle pain and spasm are the result of a primary injury to the back muscles, or a protective response to dysfunction in other spinal structures, they are symptoms common to many back pain patients.

Symptoms of Back Strain or Spasm

- intense grabbing pain
- decreased mobility
- lateral bending to the side of the spasm
- localized tenderness
- pain usually confined to the lower back, but possibly radiating to the posterior hip, groin or anterolateral thigh
- absence of neurologic signs (numbness, weakness, decreased reflexes)
- relief with rest, heat and relaxation techniques
- pain usually subsiding to dull, achy, nagging backache with diffuse distribution, resolving in 3-10 days

In some patients, muscle spasm does not resolve without intervention; the sustained contraction of the muscles can cause reduced circulation in surrounding tissue. This can initiate a cycle of pain, emotional stress, muscle tension, more spasm, more pain, etc.

Chapter 9

Muscle Strength and Back Pain

Many back experts believe that the key to a pain-free back is strong muscles; some emphasize strengthening the abdominals while others advocate physical balance among muscle groups. One of the most common philosophies in the treatment of back pain is that strengthening muscles can improve support and stability of the spine and reduce the risk of injury.

Muscles Which Affect the Spine
Abdominals

The stomach muscles flex the spine/trunk and provide the strength for such functions as coughing, straining and forced exhalation. The abdominals are composed of four individual muscles; the "rectus" runs vertically and performs straight flexion and the "obliques" run diagonally to perform flexion with rotation. [see Figure 9-1]

Good abdominal tone has long been thought to reduce stress on the spine; the need for strong abdominals has been explained in different ways.[5]

1) Abdominals balance the force of the spinal muscles that perform the opposite motion and extend the spine.

2) The oblique abdominals insert into and reinforce the fascia (connective tissue) of the spinal muscles, relieving them from the full burden of support against gravity.

3) The abdominals surround and contain the contents of the abdominal cavity; when they contract the intra-abdominal pressure created acts as an air bag that unloads pressure from the spine.

Spinal Muscles

The muscles of the spine consist of four muscle groups which attach to and connect the vertebrae. The "erector spinae" are referred to as the paravertebral, paraspinal or back extensor muscles; the fibers of this muscle group cross several vertebrae and perform the opposite motion to the abdominals - they extend the spine. [see Figure 9-1] They are responsible for maintaining an erect posture of the trunk against gravity. The strength of the extensors should normally be greater than that of the flexors, but the erector spinae have been shown to be relatively weak in people with back pain.[11]

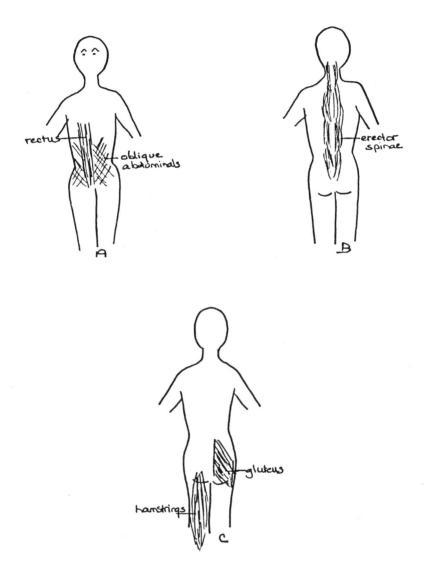

Figure 9-1. Muscles effecting the spine. (A) Abdominals (trunk flexion), front view. (B) Erector spinae (trunk extension), back view. (C) Hamstrings and gluteals (hip extension), back view.

Other smaller spinal muscles run between adjacent vertebrae. Their role is to steady the spinal column, preventing buckling between vertebrae. They provide stability at each vertebral joint, so that the erector spinae muscles can extend the whole spine in a smooth motion.[14]

Muscles Crossing the Hip Joint

The hamstring muscles participate in hip and trunk extension and the gluteal muscles participate in hip and trunk hyperextension (extension past neutral). These two muscle groups provide the power for lifting from a flexed position. The hamstrings are the muscles which form the back of the thigh; their prime action is to flex the knee. The gluteals cover the back and sides of the pelvis, forming the bulk of the buttocks; their prime actions are hip extension and abduction. [see Figure 9-1]

The hip flexor muscles assist the abdominals in trunk flexion in addition to flexing the hip joint. The bulk of the muscle is located inside the pelvis and can't easily be palpated.

The Arguments Against Muscle-Induced Back Pain

Proponents of disks, facet joints or other structures as the primary site of back pain, doubt that muscle weakness, strain or spasm could be responsible for the majority of back problems. They claim that "Spinal disorders primarily of muscular origin are uncommon."[15]

Evidence Refuting the Role of Muscles in Causing Back Pain

1) **Weakness** - The long held opinion that backache is due to weak back muscles has been discarded by some. Evidence has mounted that back musculature in humans is their most active antigravitational influence and is more than adequate to meet normal as well as extraordinary demands.[12] Strong abdominal muscles have traditionally been considered the way to protect the spine from excessive stress. However, studies show that patients with back pain do not have weak abdominals, relative to their other muscles and relative to those of people without back pain.[2,11]

A voluntary abdominal contraction is thought by many to prevent injury in flexion. However, such significant intra-abdominal pressure would be needed to neutralize the forces on the low back, (enough to interfere with abdominal circulation), that this air bag theory is questionable.[5] It is not known if a voluntary abdominal contraction can improve intra-abdominal pressure (IAP) to protect the spine; IAP is a reflex response, not a voluntary muscle contraction.[11] It is the oblique fibers of the abdominals that generate reflex intra-abdominal pressure; in a voluntary contraction the rectus is active.[11]

2) **Strain** - As with weakness, muscle strain is thought by some to be overdiagnosed, and to occur only as a result of a significant injury. Since muscles are highly vascularized and heal relatively quickly, some believe that ligament sprain versus muscle strain is responsible for the majority of prolonged back pain. When back pain keeps occurring, it may be because the ligaments have healed with weak, poorly formed scar tissue which easily re-tears again under stress.[3] Ligament sprain is consistent with the severe, localized pain which subsides to a dull, nagging, diffuse backache, common among back patients.

3) **Spasm** - Even spasm is not necessarily a primary cause of back pain, although medication is often prescribed to relieve spasm. In back patients at rest with the spine supported, EMGs show no evidence of increased muscle activity. A study which compared activity levels of spinal muscles in individuals with and without pain, found similar EMGs between the two groups. This suggests that spasm was not the primary cause of the pain.[13]

Treatment for Muscle Pathology

Acute Muscle Strain - During the early stages of an injury, rest alternated with gentle movements is advisable. Backlying with hips and knees flexed is usually the most comfortable position for resting.

Muscle Spasm - The pelvic tilt routine is an effective exercise for reducing spasm.[4] A pelvic tilt is done in backlying with hips and knees bent and feet flat on the floor or bed; the abdominals and gluteals contract to flatten the lumbar curve. Performing the motion slowly is important because a quick stretch into flexion stimulates the spastic muscle to tighten further. Application of heat is also helpful in relieving muscle spasm. The use of manipulation to reduce spasm is controversial.

Muscle Tightness - Flexibility exercises address the problem of tight back muscles; full range of motion is important for preventing muscle strain. Gentle movements should be started as soon as possible following an acute episode of pain. When stretching a muscle, a sustained position of stretch is vastly preferable to a quick stretch or to "bouncing"; these physiologically encourage the muscle to fight the stretch. All range of motion exercises should be done slowly for both protection of tissues and maximum effectiveness.

Muscle Weakness - Exercises to build both strength and endurance are recommended if back muscles are weak; both flexion and extension should be evaluated. Some patients benefit from flexion exercises and some from extension exercises and many should work for balanced strength. Muscles must become fatigued for exercises to be most effective; as a weak muscle grows stronger, more repetition or resistance is added to continue improvement. Generally, high resistance exercises build strength while repetitive exercises build endurance. Exercise should be performed slowly and done consistently, (4-7 times/week). Exercises that increase pain are probably contraindicated, while those that reduce pain are probably beneficial, contradicting the "no pain, no gain" philosophy.[6]

Tension - Muscular and emotional tension often coexist. Relaxation techniques are used to reduce tension and are often incorporated into other treatment programs. They may be used to decrease muscle spasm or stretch tight muscles. Other types of relaxation training reduce anxiety and improve a patient's sense of control; patients are encouraged to gain mental mastery over their tension. Many programs emphasize the importance of combining physical and mental relaxation. Examples are breathing exercises, visualization, hypnosis, biofeedback, massage and Yoga.

Poor Use of Muscles - The way the body is positioned in sitting, sleeping, lifting and moving has a strong impact on the health of the back. "Posture and Body Mechanics" is covered in Chapter 13 and is a recommended part of any treatment approach to back pain. Some exercise programs emphasize movement reeducation to correct pain-induced abnormal movement patterns.

Myofascial Restrictions - The importance of fascial tightening as a cause of pain is the focus of several controversial treatment approaches. These include myofascial release and cranio-sacral therapy. Manipulation of fascial restrictions and of the bones of the skull and sacrum is performed. This is thought to restore normal alignment, energy flow, soft tissue mobility and even to free unresolved emotions.

Trigger Points - Trigger point therapy aims at achieving restoration of full muscle length and strength. Techniques used to deactivate trigger points include massage, injection and deep pressure directly on the site. (Specific methods are listed in Chapter 12, "Piriformis Syndrome".) These may be followed by heat, range of motion exercises and relaxation techniques.

A booklet on pain put out in 1953 states that most back and neck pain patients, with their "exaggerated sense of responsibility", drive themselves beyond their endurance, suffering general fatigue which produces nervous and muscular tension states.[10] Adequate rest is recommended. The back pain booklets published for laymen today no longer emphasize nervous energy and rest; instead they encourage "strong flexible muscles to support the back's natural, balanced position".[8]

That the spinal muscles are an important factor in back pain is unquestionable. However, concluding that "most" back pain is a result of tension or weakness is surely an over-simplification; the "National Back Fitness Test" is an example. This program promises to "show you the common exercises that will help you prevent backache for the rest of your life" and claims that those with a good score are the least likely to suffer a back problem.[9] From a possible score of 4 (the best) to 16 (the worst), this author (who suffers from chronic disabling back pain) got a 5!

Key Points - Strains, Sprains and Spasms

One of the most common approaches in the treatment of back pain is to strengthen the abdominal and back extensor muscles. Not only weakness, but also tightness, tension, spasm or postural fatigue have each been considered to be the cause of most back problems. Critics argue that weakness, strain and spasm are unlikely to be primary causes of back pain. The muscles that support the back play a role in an injury-free spine, but concluding that weak or tense muscles explain most back pain is an oversimplification.

Footnotes

1 Edward Abraham, *Freedom from Back Pain: An Orthopedist's Self-Help Guide*
2 Glenna Batson, "Reeducating or Strengthening: Relooking at the Pelvic Tilt"
3 Ben Benjamin, "The Mystery of Lower Back Pain"

Chapter 9

4 Blackburn & Portney, "Electromyographic Activity of Back Musculature During Williams Flexion Exercises"
5 Rene Cailliet, *Low Back Pain Syndrome*
6 Deborah Caplan, *Back Trouble*
7 Charles Fager, "Facts and Fallacies of Spinal Disorders: A Neurosurgeon's Viewpoint"
8 Nancy Friedman, "Back Exercises for a Healthy Back"
9 David Imrie, *Goodbye Back Ache*
10 Ishmael & Shorbe, "Care of the Back"
11 Jackson & Brown, "Analysis of Current Approaches and a Practical Guide to Prescription of Exercise"
12 George Lawn, "How to Lift - Is There a Right Way?"
13 David Miller, "Comparison of Electromyographic Activity in the Lumbar Paraspinal Muscle of Subjects with and without Low Back Pain"
14 Stanley Paris, "Physical Signs of Instability"
15 Duane Saunders, *Evaluation, Treatment and Prevention of Musculoskeletal Disorders*
16 Michael Shea, "MFR and the Psychosomatic Body"
17 Simons & Travell, "Myofascial Origins of Low Back Pain"
18 Muhammed Yunus, "Primary Fibromyalgia"

Chapter 10 - Spondylosis

"The majority of chronic, disabling low back pain is due to degenerative changes." Bernard Jacobs, MD[5] / *"Back pain is most commonly due to arthritis affecting the back by narrowing the disks."* George Lewith, MD & Sandra Horn[7]

"Degenerative changes of the joints are commonly asymptomatic." Paul Kaplan, MD & Ellen Tanner, PT[6] / "The percentage of patients with back pain does not progress with age or correlate with degenerative changes." Rene Cailliet, MD[2]

Degenerative changes of the spine involve narrowing of disks, flattening of the vertebral bodies, facet joint wear and tear and soft tissue changes; in some cases bone spurs grow and nerves are pinched. [see Figure 10-1] The combination of these changes is called "spondylosis," literally a condition affecting vertebrae. This is what is meant when patients are told they have degenerative disease of the spine, arthritis of the spine or degenerative disk disease. These changes alter the spine's balance, predisposing it to secondary injury.

However, the extent of the apparent damage does not necessarily correspond to pain felt. Spondylosis is the most common x-ray finding in older patients and shouldn't be considered the cause of pain before all other causes are excluded.[3] By the fifth decade, 90 percent of men and 60 percent of

A

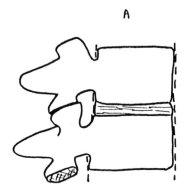

B

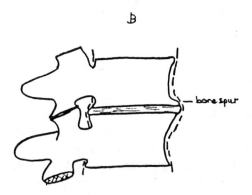

Figure 10-1. (A) Section of the spinal column showing two vertebrae, side view. (B) Spondylosis of spinal column, (flattened and misshapen vertebral bodies, flattened disks, worn down and jammed facet joints, narrowed spinal canal, stretched ligaments and development of bone spurs.)

women show x-ray evidence of spondylosis.[8] Even bone spurs do not necessarily produce pain; they are present on x-ray in 41 percent of men and 27 percent of women between ages 55-64 in the cervical region and 23 percent of men and 13 percent of women in the lumbar region.[1]

The Structural Changes of Aging
- weakening and tearing of the outer annular fibers of the disks
- shrunken and sometimes prolapsed disks which no longer correctly attach, restrain, space and position vertebrae
- reduction in water content of the nucleus of disks, which impairs redistribution of spinal pressure
- thinning and cracking of the vertebral body's surfaces, which allows shearing of vertebrae
- thinning of bones (osteoporosis) and development of bone spurs
- increased laxity of ligaments
- loss of support from the longitudinal ligaments
- arthritic changes in facet joints with compression of the joint surfaces and thickening of the joint capsules
- narrowing of the spinal canal, called "stenosis"
- asymmetric disk degeneration causing a lateral spinal curvature of individual spinal segments called "tropism"
- a torque (twisting force) caused by the tropism, with the facet on the concave side compressing and the facet on the convex side subluxing

The Postural Changes of Aging
- loss of muscle tone and postural sagging with exaggerated spinal curves
- vertebrae and disks being pulled out of alignment, stressing the weaker areas of the spine
- loss of range of motion with shortening of muscles and ligaments
- weakening of the whole spinal structure, predisposing it to injury

Spinal deterioration is caused by chemical and physical changes that start to develop during late adolescence; it is the result of physiological aging plus mechanical stress. Spondylosis is a natural process of aging, often painless, but may also develop prematurely. Some feel early degenerative changes have an auto-immune basis.[5] Mechanically, spondylosis can be hastened by reduced or by excessive range of motion. Hypomobility can speed degenerative changes due to a decreased blood supply; hypermobility can produce the same end result from a variety of causes - poor posture, congenital defects, trauma or overtreatment by manipulation or stretching. Degenerative changes occur in everyone and it is unknown why they are painful and disabling in only certain people.

Manipulation is not helpful in the diagnosis of spondylosis, while myelography and CAT scans often are. Radiographic studies may show the following.
- bone spurs
- spinal stenosis (narrowing of the spinal canal)
- flattening of the surfaces of the vertebral bodies
- thickening, shortening or overlapping of the bones which form the arch of a vertebra
- degeneration of facet joints

Common Symptoms of Spondylosis
- age of patients usually 50 or older
- gradual onset with a history of back pain
- pain occurring in cycles with pain-free months or years
- dull aching in the low back and hips, with possible sciatica or aching into the legs
- sitting more comfortable than standing
- pain aggravated by standing for long periods
- pain worse in morning and evening, especially upon rising
- stiffness and limitation in range of motion, especially extension
- feelings of weakness in the legs
- radiating pain or neurologic signs from spinal stenosis, which subside after sitting
- some loss of the lumbar lordosis
- with tropism (asymmetrical disk degeneration), pain especially severe on extension with simultaneous lateral flexion toward the concave side

Radiating pain and neurologic signs from a disk rupture are aggravated by flexion. In contrast, flexion relieves these symptoms with spondylosis; flexion lengthens the spinal canal, separates facet joints and increases circulatory capacity.[2]

Treatment for Spondylosis

Although it is not possible to reverse the changes of aging, there are a variety of treatments for spondylosis which provide symptomatic relief or which correct the mechanisms which may speed degeneration.

1) use of proper posture and body mechanics to reduce stress on the spine

2) mobility exercises to prevent further loss of range of motion and improve circulation

3) avoidance of hyperextension (arching the trunk past a neutral position) and of stomach-lying to reduce compression of facet joint surfaces

4) heat and aspirin for symptomatic relief of achiness

5) use of ice during acute flare-ups to reduce inflammation

6) therapy comprising gentle flexion-rotation mobilization techniques to improve mobility and inhibit pain

7) epidural injection, (injection of a steroid into the area surrounding the spinal cord and nerve roots), when stenosis is causing pain due to nerve root compression

8) surgery in cases where a bone spur or stenosis is causing nerve root compression with severe pain and neurologic signs

Spondylosis has a variety of components, any one of which can cause back pain directly or through secondary changes. Regardless of x-ray abnormalities, spondylosis may also be, and frequently is, asymptomatic. A diagnosis of arthritis or degenerative disease carries with it a sense of hopelessness and fear of ever-increasing disability. Such a diagnosis may have no relevance to a patient's pain or the ability to treat it.

Key Points - Spondylosis

Spondylosis is a condition which involves degenerative changes of spinal structures; vertebrae and disks flatten, facet joints are compressed and soft tissues are stretched. These changes may be painful or may make the spine susceptible to other injuries. However, spondylosis is a normal component of aging and usually the degenerative changes seen on x-ray are asymptomatic. When spondylosis produces pain and neurologic signs, symptomatic treatment is available. Patients can also make life-style changes which may slow down the degenerative process.

Footnotes

1   American Medical Association, *Book of Back Care*
2   Rene Cailliet, *Low Back Pain Syndrome*
3   CIBA, "Low Back Pain"
4   Charles Fager, "The Neurosurgical Management of Lumbar Spine Disease"
5   Bernard Jacobs, "Low Back Pain: The Orthopedist's View"
6   Kaplan & Tanner, *Musculoskeletal Pain and Disability*
7   Lewith & Horn, *Drug Free Pain Relief*
8   John Rice, et al., "Low Back Pain: The Rheumatologist's View"

Chapter 11 - Sacro-Iliac Joint Dysfunction

"In evaluation of patients with low back pain, our most frequent finding is the presence of a sacro-iliac joint dysfunction." Michael Cibulka, PT, and Rhonda Koldehoff, PT[6] / *"Of all cases with pain in the low back referred to this department, just over 80 percent have anterior dysfunction of the sacro-iliac joint."* Richard DonTigny, PT[8]

"I have come slowly to the conclusion that displacements of the sacrum on the ilium [sacro-iliac joint dysfunction] *do not occur."* James Cyriax, MD[7]

The sacro-iliac joints (SIJs) connect the sides of the sacrum to the part of the pelvis called the ilium (plural: ilia). [see Figure 11-1] Before disk pathology was recognized in the 1930s, the sacro-iliac joint was considered a primary site of back pain. SIJ dysfunction then fell out of favor as a diagnosis and some practitioners still believe SI joint displacements do not occur. What makes evaluation difficult is a symptomatology of back, buttock, leg, hip and/or groin pain which is similar to that found with other low back pain syndromes. Sacro-iliac joint dysfunction (SIJD) may also co-exist with lumbar and hip problems, further confusing the diagnosis.

The sacro-iliac is an extremely stable joint due to powerful supporting ligaments, but one with no direct muscular support. Normally the stiff, inelastic ligaments prevent excessive or abnormal movement; in fact, no joint movement can be noted on x-ray, (an argument for the non-existence of SIJ

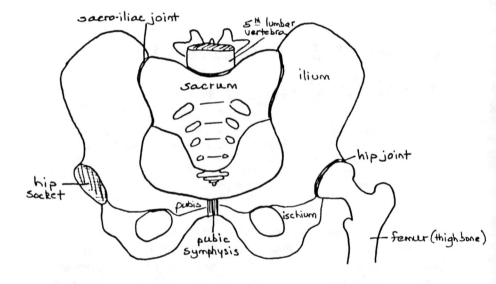

Figure 11-1. The pelvis and sacrum, front view.

displacement). However, the sacro-iliac joint can be affected by sprains, inflammation, hypomobility, hypermobility, subluxations or degenerative joint disease just like any other synovial joint. Most now agree the joint does move, but as its motion is variable and limited, the degree and direction of movement are controversial.[11] To complicate the understanding of this joint, irregularities in the SIJ begin developing after puberty and variations in the anatomy of the joint surface exist among individuals. [see Box 11-1]

Normal Movement of the Sacro-Iliac Joint

1) The greatest movement occurs as rotation around a transverse (left-right) axis during flexion and extension of the lumbar spine. At the end of the range in forward flexion, the wedge-shaped sacrum causes gapping of the ilia away from the sacrum.

2) Linear displacement also occurs at the end of the range in trunk flexion; the sacrum slides vertically in an upslip or downslip.[3]

3) One-sided or asymmetrical SIJ motion is accompanied by movement of the pubic symphysis, (the fibrous joint at the front of the pelvis). It occurs during lateral flexion or rotation of the lumbar spine and during one-sided or opposing hip movements. The sacrum follows the same direction of lateral flexion and rotation as the spine.[3,4]

4) Slight rotation around a horizontal (front to back) or vertical axis may exist in combination with the vertical slip of the sacrum.[3]

Box 11-1

Abnormal joint movement may be excessive (hypermobility) or restricted (hypomobility). SIJ hypomobility is probably age-related and asymptomatic; however, if the joint is very loose it may override its normal boundary and become stuck, appearing hypomobile when the opposite is true.[10] In an individual with exaggerated spinal curves, the sacrum lies more horizontal and is quite mobile. At the limits of its small range, no great force is needed to damage the ligaments of the SIJ, causing instability.[12] Hypermobility probably predisposes the joint to sprain and entrapment.[11,14] [see Box 11-2]

Abnormal Movement of the Sacro-Iliac Joint

The most common type of sacro-iliac joint dysfunction, an "anterior dysfunction," frequently occurs during trunk flexion in standing, with inadequate support of the anterior pelvis from the abdominals. The ilia rotate anteriorly and down relative to the sacrum. Because the strong posterior ligaments are on slack in the flexed position and because the sacrum is wider anteriorly, the sacrum tends to spread the ilia; this gapping allows the sacrum to become trapped.[9] This stretches the joint capsule causing acute pain. The resultant downward/posterior position of the hip joint relative to the sacrum causes an apparent leg lengthening; this puts the spinal nerve roots on stretch, often causing inflammation and sciatica. A further complication can occur when, after the ilia rotate anteriorly, they also slip vertically upward on the sacrum and lock.[9] More common bilaterally (55 percent),[8] anterior SIJD also occurs on one side, causing asymmetry in the positioning of the pelvis.

Box 11-2

Causes of SIJD

Possible causes of sacro-iliac joint dysfunction are many and include the following:

- trauma to the pelvis or sacrum
- childbirth and multiple pregnancies
- musculoskeletal diseases
- abnormal gait or posture
- hypermobility of joints and an exaggerated lumbar curve
- occupational stresses affecting the pelvis
- leg length differences of as little as 1/4 inch
- injuries of the legs or spine
- lateral curvature of the spine
- spasm of the piriformis muscle

Some consider the most common cause of SIJD to be an imbalance (of at least 15 percent) in length or strength of the muscle groups active in normal pelvic alignment. Asymmetry may be between left and right sides or between a muscle and its antagonist, (the muscle performing the opposite motion). Hip external rotation-internal rotation imbalance is especially common.[6]

Another view of SIJD puts the blame for back, hip and leg pain directly on the sacral ligaments. These massive, crisscrossing ligaments can be strained in may ways and in dozens of places. Sacral movements can create either a pinching or a shearing stress; even poor posture or muscle imbalance can cause repeated strains to the ligaments, with scar tissue build-up.[5]

Diagnosis

Pain is the primary symptom of SIJD, affecting the joint itself and often buttock, hip and leg. Pain is aggravated by prolonged or repetitive postures or activities; these include. . .

- weight-bearing positions (pain relieved by movement),
- combined hip and trunk flexion,
- combined hip and trunk extension, or
- flexion of one hip with extension of the other.

Diagnosing SIJD is not straight-forward; different studies show conflicting degrees of reliability for specific tests.

Subjective guidelines are based on the patient's pain and are heavily relied upon; they may be the most statistically reliable.[13] Objective testing is done by palpating the bony landmarks of the pelvis during movement and noting asymmetries; asymmetry in soft tissue tension and joint play are also noted. The apparent leg lengthening caused by the downward movement of the hip socket relative to the SI joint is a useful indicator in diagnosis. [see Box 11-3]

Clinical Tests for SIJD

Pain-based tests are as follows:

- tenderness over the SIJ
- tenderness over the pubic symphysis
- tenderness over the crest of the ilium
- pain on compression of the SIJ (in backlying or sidelying)
- pain on resisted hip abduction with hip extended
- presence of SIJ pain on the side of the high pubis
- pain with gapping of the ilia, (a possible cause of pain in sitting)
- pain with both forward and backward torsion strain (suspect hypermobility)
- pain with either forward or backward torsion strain (suspect entrapment)
- presence of SIJ pain on opposite side of straight leg raise (SLR) or absence of pain on same side of SLR

Tests for asymmetry or for limitations of pelvic mobility include the following:

- reduced mobility in the SIJ
- reduced spring in the SIJ
- disruption of the pubic symphysis
- uneven iliac crests and PSISs,* with level ASISs* and trochanters*
- failure of PSISs* to drop while marching in place
- lower PSIS* becoming higher during forward flexion
- apparent leg lengthening (measured from PSIS* to medial malleolus)
- appearance of leg length discrepancy as patient comes from backlying to long-sitting
- disappearance of above sign following manipulation of the SIJ to correct the dysfunction.

* The ASIS and PSIS are bony landmarks on the pelvis; trochanters are prominences on the femur, or thigh bone.

Box 11-3

Treatment for Sacro-Iliac Joint Dysfunction

1) **Rest** - Acute inflammation of the SI joint may require a short period of bedrest. For this initial period the preferred positions are (1) backlying with a pillow under the edge of the buttocks or (2) sidelying with a pillow between the knees and the lower leg relatively extended; the pillow keeps the spine from twisting and the top leg from slipping forward. Rest should be alternated with gentle activity.

2) **Manipulation** - Manipulation is by far the most widely recommended approach for treating SIJD; some studies show over 90 percent of patients responding positively.[2,11]   Although the entrapped joint may respond dramatically to manipulation which restores movement, the result can be a return to hypermobility with its associated pain and a tendency to reoccurrence.[10] Manipulation can also aggravate the condition if it is not specific for an SIJ dysfunction. [see Box 11-4]

Manipulation for Sacro-Iliac Joint Dysfunction
The indication for SIJ manipulation is strong if the leg length discrepancy test is positive and if force in the opposite direction of the suspected entrapment reduces pain. With an anterior dysfunction, manipulation is accomplished by vigorously rotating the ilium posteriorly on the sacrum. This should be preceded by traction if a vertical slip complicates the dysfunction. If ligamentous sprain is present, manipulation may help by relieving stress on the sacral ligaments or by tearing weakened fibers to allow stronger healing.[5]

Manipulation must consist of a maneuver to specifically correct SIJD, versus a spinal adjustment. The traditional manipulative approach to treating a high iliac crest has been to extend the ilium on the sacrum in the mistaken belief that the high crest is caused by an upward versus an anterior dysfunction. This maneuver can separate the joint, allowing the ligaments to rebound the ilium into place for immediate relief; if done repeatedly, however, it increases instability.[8]

Box 11-4

---

3) **Bracing** - Because the sacrum is not supported muscularly, it may be necessary to use a mechanical support following correction by manipulation. A "trochanteric belt with a sacral pad" is used to maintain alignment. It consists of a small pad which sits directly over the sacrum; it is held on by a strap which goes over the hip joints. Such support may have to be long-term with chronic instability, obesity or very weak abdominals.

4) **Exercise** - Support should be provided to the anterior pelvis through abdominal strengthening exercises. It is thought that a strong contraction of the abdominals can prevent anterior dysfunction during forward bending.[9] Stretching tight muscles is also recommended, including the piriformis muscles and hip flexors. Correcting muscle tightness can reportedly improve SIJ imbalance in 60 percent of patients.[1]

5) **Injections** - "Proliferant" injections into affected sacroiliac ligaments are considered by some to be a very effective treatment in the long run.[5] The proliferant causes an inflammatory response leading to the production of new ligamentous tissue.[12] The injections promote healing and strengthening of the ligaments with the goal of preventing a recurrence of SIJD by increasing joint stability. A series of injections is required.

Sacro-iliac joint dysfunction is probably the most complicated of the low back syndromes to understand, diagnose and treat. The joint itself is difficult to visualize with its limited and controversial range of motion; practitioners need to be familiar with the specifics of evaluation and manipulation which are unique to this affliction. Experts on SIJ dysfunction believe that practitioners are just coming to realize how pervasive it is. Appropriate intervention is not only important to relieve pain, but if untreated, the condition can lead to degenerative problems, especially involving the head of the femur (thigh bone) and the L-5/S-1 disk.[9]

Key Points - Sacro-Iliac Joint Dysfunction

The sacro-iliac joint is a very stable joint with strong ligaments for support. Its movement is variable and limited and therefore controversial. SIJ dysfunction occurs most commonly when the sacrum becomes entrapped by the pelvis during trunk flexion. It causes pain over the joint and often in the buttock, hip and leg. Diagnosis of SIJD depends on subjective testing of the location of pain and what aggravates it. Asymmetry of bony landmarks and limitations in pelvic mobility are also used for diagnosis. The most effective treatment is considered to be manipulation to correct the entrapment. SIJD requires specialized training on the part of the practitioner; its specific diagnostic and treatment techniques are unique to this affliction.

Footnotes

1 "Approaches to Musculoskeletal Problems: Focus on the Low Back" Symposium, Michael Irwin
2 *The Back Letter*, Vol. 4, No. 2
3 Myron Beal, "The Sacroiliac Problem: Review of Anatomy, Mechanics and Diagnosis"
4 Nicholas Bellamy, et al., "What Do We Know About the Sacroiliac Joint?"
5 Ben Benjamin, "The Mystery of Lower Back Pain"
6 Cibulka & Koldehoff, "Evaluating Chronic Sacroiliac Joint Dysfunction"
7 James Cyriax, *Textbook of Orthopaedic Medicine*
8 Richard DonTigny, "Dysfunction of the Sacroiliac Joint and Its Treatment"
9 Richard DonTigny, "Function and Pathomechanics of the Sacroiliac Joint"
10 Elizabeth Grieve, "Lumbo-pelvic Rhythm and Mechanical Dysfunction of the Sacro-Iliac Joint."
11 McGregor & Cassidy, "Post-surgical Sacroiliac Joint Syndrome"
12 Milne Ongley, et al., "A New Approach to the Treatment of Chronic Back Pain"
13 Potter & Rothstein, "Intertester Reliability for Selected Clinical Tests of the Sacroiliac Joint"
14 Duane Saunders, *Evaluation, Treatment and Prevention of Musculoskeletal Disorders*

Chapter 12 - Piriformis Syndrome

"One of the causes of failed back surgery is the 'pyriformis syndrome'." Ricky Lockett, PT[3]

"Apologists have put forward the alternative of spasm of the piriformis muscle, but if this actually happened, the hip would be fixed in full abduction, and it is not." James Cyriax, MD[2]

The piriformis muscle lies within the pelvis, connecting the sacrum to the top of the thigh bone. Its main action is to externally rotate the hip; it abducts and extends the hip as well. The large sciatic nerve, which runs down the back of the thigh, leaves the pelvis at mid-buttock, directly below or even through the middle of the piriformis. [see Figure 12-1] The theory behind the pirifomis syndrome is that pain is caused by the sciatic nerve becoming compressed by spasm of the piriformis muscle.[1]

When the lumbar spine is stressed by weak musculature or trauma, protective spasm of the piriformis may occur in an attempt to stabilize the area. This puts pressure on the nerve and causes symptoms similar to that of lumbar disk disease. Sacro-iliac joint dysfunction may also cause piriformis spasm.

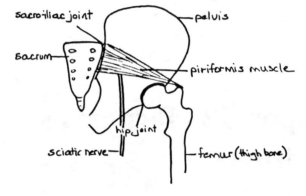

Figure 12-1. Pelvis, sacrum and thigh bone, back view, with piriformis muscle and sciatic nerve.

Symptoms of Piriformis Syndrome

- pain and/or paresthesia (abnormal sensation) in buttock, SI joint, hip and along the path of the sciatic nerve ("sciatica")
- tender points at the muscle's origin or insertion
- increased discomfort with active hip external rotation (ER) or passive internal rotation (IR)
- decreased active and passive hip IR
- positioning of the hip in ER in backlying
- increased pain, paresthesia or spasm upon palpation of the muscle
- absence of neurologic signs

Sciatica is also a common symptom of a disk rupture. Differentiating piriformis syndrome from disk rupture is determined with a straight leg raise. With piriformis syndrome, the SLR is initially negative or produces only mild sciatic pain; the SLR becomes positive by incorporating forceful hip internal rotation. Injection of an anesthetic agent directly into the muscle is also diagnostic.[1]

Treatment of Piriformis Syndrome

Treatment of the piriformis syndrome is aimed first at minimizing the muscle spasm to restore blood flow and reduce pain. This is followed by stretch to lengthen the muscle and relieve pressure on the sciatic nerve. Sustained relief also requires resolution of the factors which initiated piriformis spasm.

Treatment Techniques

- muscle inhibition techniques to relax the muscle for optimum stretch
- "spray and stretch" (muscle stretching preceded by a vapocoolant spray to inhibit pain and spasm)
- icing, high voltage galvanic stimulation, ultra-sound or other physical agents that inhibit muscle spasm; followed by stretch
- "trigger point deactivation"; deep manual pressure on the most painful site of the muscle to block circulation, denying oxygen to the area
- vaginal or rectal massage of the muscle
- steroid injection into the muscle belly (vaginal injection preferred)
- surgical cutting of the muscle

The interrelatedness of the structures of the spine make piriformis spasm a possible offshoot of other low back syndromes. Some also believe that piriformis syndrome plays a more significant role than most practitioners realize in initiating back pain.

Key Points - Piriformis Syndrome

The piriformis syndrome results when the sciatic nerve is compressed by a spasm of the piriformis muscle. The symptoms include pain and paresthesia in the buttock, sacro-iliac joint, hip and along the sciatic nerve distribution. Treatment involves relieving spasm in the muscle, followed by stretch to reduce pressure on the sciatic nerve.

Footnotes

1 Rene Cailliet, *Low Back Pain Syndrome*
2 James Cyriax, *Textbook of Orthopaedic Medicine*
3 Ricky Lockett, "Pyriformis Syndrome - Diagnosis and Treatment"

Chapter 13 - The Role of Posture in Back Pain

"The spine is poorly designed for standing erect." Philip Gildenberg & Richard DeVaul[2]
"Back problems are often due to excessive sitting in our society." James McGavin, PT[5]
"If you have chronic low back pain, the blame probably lies with the way you use your back." Deborah Caplan[1]

Posture is the position one assumes against gravity; body mechanics is the posture of the body in motion. The goal of good posture is to maintain balanced alignment against gravity with the minimum use of energy. The spine has four continuous curves for flexibility and shock absorption; energy efficient posture requires that the normal curves are maintained to put the muscles at optimum working length. [see Figure 13-1] The spinal column is supported by a complex system of muscles, ligaments and joints, all working together. Ligamentous support occurs without energy expenditure; muscle action intervenes at the limits of ligament stress. Poor posture causes reduced efficiency in the skeletal/ligament systems; a prolonged position of poor posture, with flattened or exaggerated curves, overstretches and overworks the muscles. For example, the neck supports the weight of the head, normally 8-12 pounds. When an individual sits with the head hanging forward, a torque is created at the base of the neck, increasing the force of the head on the neck to as much as 36 pounds.[7]

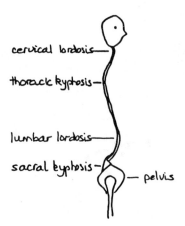

Figure 13-1. Correct standing posture, side view, characterized by the maintenance of the natural curves of the spine.

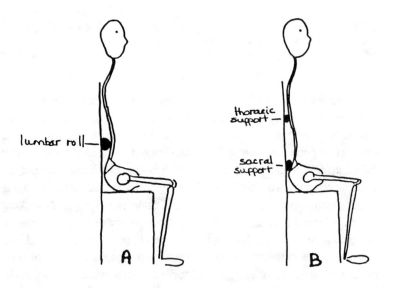

Figure 13-2. (A) Use of a lumbar roll in sitting to maintain a lumbar lordosis. (B) Use of a thoracic and sacral support for spinal stability in sitting.

As people grow older, changes occur which are probably due more to lifestyle than physiological aging. The muscles lose tone and become deconditioned. The head juts forward, shoulders sag, chest sinks, butt and abdomen protrude and the spinal curves increase. Flexibility and range of motion are lost; muscles, tendons and ligaments shorten. With an increasingly slouched posture, added stress is put on muscles and spinal structures, so that vertebrae and disks are pulled out of their normal alignment. The whole spinal structure becomes weakened and more vulnerable to injury. When pain is suddenly elicited during a specific incident, the assumption is often made that something has slipped out of place or snapped. Most back and neck problems, however, are probably not caused by a single injury; a healthy back is unlikely to be hurt by a single twist, lift or fall.[8] Much more commonly, symptoms are the result of months or years of stress to the spine from poor posture, faulty body mechanics, stressful working and living habits, loss of flexibility and general decline of physical fitness.[6]

Poor posture is a possible cause of or contributing factor toward dysfunction in any spinal structure. Proper posture and body mechanics is one of the few treatment approaches which is advised for virtually every person with back pain, as well as for prevention. No treatment can undo the harmful effects of continual misuse of the back, but it is never too late to learn how to stand, sit, bend, lift and sleep correctly.

Treatment to Improve Posture and Body Mechanics

Adjusting the body's posture and movement, unlike treatments such as manipulation or surgery, is one of the few approaches which is universally helpful for every back pain patient. Part of a rehabilitation program for back pain should include an individualized assessment of posture and body mechanics. Many Physical Therapy departments offer "Back School," a class to teach proper use of the back. Patients then need to make these new habits permanent.

For many years, flattening the lumbar lordosis through the "pelvic tilt routine" was considered the appropriate approach for protecting the back. This is no longer a universal recommendation:

"Good posture hinges on the pelvic tilt." David Imrie, MD[3] / *"Avoid swayback at all times."* William Ishmael, MD & Howard Shorbe, MD[4]

"The usual recommendation to pelvic tilt is bad for the spine as it

prevents free use of the hip joint, increasing strain on the lower back, and keeps the spine from efficient vertical alignment." Deborah Caplan[1]

Most specialists now recommend maintenance of the natural, gentle curves of neck and back during all activities; a degree of lordosis is encouraged as desirable and physiologically sound. Eliminating lordosis by flattening or bowing out the lower back overstretches soft tissues and increases pressure on the disks. Excessive lordosis also stresses the back, especially those structures at the apex of the curve. These effects are exaggerated by obesity which further increases the curve and adds wear and tear on the joints and disks. Part of a posture program includes the recommendation for weight loss, if appropriate.

General guidelines for good posture and body mechanics include the following:

- Maintain the balanced position of your back, (with natural curves), for all activities.
- Change position frequently to unload joints, relax muscles and redistribute pressure on weight-bearing surfaces.
- Minimize bending and twisting at the same time.
- Have your work surface close to you in order to avoid bending forward.
- Split up tasks into enough steps to avoid unbalanced positions or excessive strain.
- After periods of prolonged sitting or driving, walk around and stretch into extension; avoid bending or lifting until your back has had time to recover.
- Ask for help when necessary; ask yourself if it's really necessary to do this activity!

Everything said about faulty posture and body mechanics applies to necks as well as low backs. As with low backs, the goal for reducing neck pain is balanced alignment and maintenance of the normal spinal curves. Line up the ear with the shoulder, have work at the proper height, change positions of the neck frequently, lift correctly, etc.

The person with back pain often has to take extra measures to find a comfortable position and to reduce stress on spinal structures. She may have to find new ways of lifting. [see Figure 13-3] He may have to use special

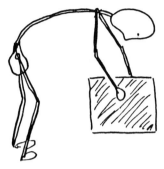

Figure 13-3. Lifting with a flattened lumbar spine which increases stress on the disks.

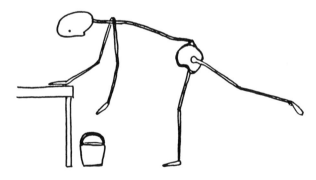

Golfer's lift which maintains the natural curves of the spine during forward bending.

119

equipment for sitting and driving. [see Figure 13-2] There are excellent guides for posture and body mechanics for people with all levels of back pain. Many are inexpensive and well worth reading and applying so that the spine won't continue to be subjected to repeated injury and stress through improper use. *Managing Back Pain, For Your Neck, Sex and Back Pain* and other booklets are available from Educational Opportunities in Bloomington, Minnesota; call 1-800-654-8357 for a catalog.

Key Points - Posture and Body Mechanics

Using proper posture and body mechanics is recommended for everybody - for minimizing back pain, preventing its occurrence or reoccurrence and for giving other treatment approaches the best chance for success. The postural changes associated with aging weaken the entire spinal structure and make the back more vulnerable to injury; years of preventable abuse may cause many back and neck problems. It is never too late to learn to reduce the harmful effects caused by continual misuse of the back.

Footnotes

1   Deborah Caplan, *Back Trouble*
2   Gildenberg & DeVaul, *The Chronic Pain Patient*
3   David Imrie, *Goodbye Back Ache*
4   Ishmael & Shorbe, "Care of the Back"
5   James McGavin, "The McKenzie Approach to Spinal Pain"
6   Melnick, et al., *Managing Back Pain*
7   Paulette Olsen, "Brief Media Presentation on Back Care"
8   Duane Saunders, *The Back Care Program*

Chapter 14 - Author's Recommendations

"...advice is a dangerous gift, even from the wise to the wise, and all courses may run ill."
J.R.R. Tolkien, *The Fellowship of the Ring*

Comments Concerning Diagnosis and Treatment

The diagnoses and diagnostic rationales discussed in *The Diagnosis and Misdiagnosis of Back Pain* have critics as well as avid proponents. This reinforces the fact that every explanation for back pain is appropriate for some patients, but not one is the answer for everyone. The premise of this book reflects the confusion and controversy surrounding this condition; it is that **the diagnosis and treatment of back pain must be individualized.**

Unfortunately, many people assume that "most" patients with back pain have the same problem and require the same type of intervention. The following diagnoses and treatments are appropriate and successful for some patients, but they are too often applied indiscriminately. Practitioners who are too committed to a philosophy tend to blame the patient if the treatment is unsuccessful. [see Box 14-1]

One-Size-Fits-All Approaches to Back Pain

Diagnosis	Practitioner	Treatment
somatic dysfunction	osteopath	manipulation
vertebral subluxation	chiropractor	spinal adjustment
back strain	MD	bedrest, heat, medications, corset
arthritis	MD	symptomatic treatment
weak abdominals	any & all	flexion exercises
stress/tension	any & all	relaxation techniques, counseling

Practitioners of many alternative approaches, (spiritual healing, Rolfing, foot reflexology, myofascial release, Feldenkrais, acupuncture and macrobiotics, to name just a few), may regard all back pain as the result of a single factor. The presumed causes include blocked energy, fascial restrictions, unresolved emotions, tension, poor nutrition or negative feelings.

Box 14-1

Health professionals with expertise in tailoring exercises to the individual back pain patient include physiatrists, (MDs specializing in rehabilitation and physical medicine), physical therapists and sports medicine doctors. Other practitioners who can individualize exercise programs include kinesiologists, (experts in the principles and mechanics of movement), and Yoga or physical fitness instructors with special training in back dysfunction.[1]

Recommendations for People with Back Pain

Despite variation and controversy in the diagnosis and treatment of back pain, there are some general guidelines which can be applied to every back problem. The following recommendations are meant for anyone with back pain; like all advice, apply it judiciously to your own situation.

Diagnosis
1) Become informed about backs and what can happen to them.
2) Find a health care professional with whom you can communicate and

work together to understand and treat your back pain. Ask about the rationale of various treatments in order to avoid having unrealistic expectations.

3) Don't assume that you can be your own diagnostician. Your input is valuable, but you cannot evaluate all the subtleties of movement dysfunction that a qualified practitioner can.

4) Remember that a list of symptoms in a book serves only as a general guideline. Every person is unique, as is every back problem.

Treatment

1) Keep bedrest to a minimum; a maximum of two days is now considered sufficient for most acute episodes. Alternate bedrest with a brief period of moving about every one to two hours.

2) Both performing pelvic tilts and the application of heat can be effective in relieving muscle spasm. However, during the first 24-48 hours following an episode of acute pain, try using ice instead of heat; it is considered preferable for the reduction of inflammation.

3) Minimize your use of medications, especially on a long-term basis.

4) Avoid surgery as a cure for pain; there are very clear and limited conditions for which surgery is appropriate.

5) There is evidence that vigorous manipulation has no advantage over mobilization techniques; the gentlest kind of manual therapy which is effective is recommended. If manipulation is the appropriate treatment for your condition, there should be significant improvement in pain or mobility within 3 treatments.

6) Whether on bedrest, working, driving or relaxing, change position frequently. Immobility is bad for backs.

7) If you were injured on the job, a rehabilitation program that simulates your work place can speed your return to work; discuss a referral to a "Work Hardening" program with your doctor.

8) A back condition requires the right balance of rest, activity and common sense. Listen to your body; society may place a premium on being tough, but a "no pain, no gain" approach is overrated.

9) Consider the role of stress or tension in your back pain and don't be afraid to incorporate relaxation techniques or counseling as one component of your overall treatment program. However, if your practitioner automatically assumes your pain is emotionally based and you disagree, feel free to seek a second opinion.

10) There is much talk about the use of positive thought to cure health problems. Without question, a positive attitude and sense of humor improve the quality of your life; they may do much more. However, they are unable to cure everyone's back pain. If a treatment approach is unsuccessful, don't assume it's because you didn't try hard enough.

There are few approaches without critics, but the following seem to be universally recommended. For pain reduction as well as prevention they should be incorporated into your daily routine for the rest of your life.

- good posture and body mechanics
- a physical conditioning program suited to your level of functioning
- attention to your overall health needs
- taking responsibility for the management of your back pain

Recommended Reading

Lauren Hebert, *Sex and Back Pain* (a practical guide for finding comfortable positions for sex)

Barbara Headley, *Chronic Pain: Life Out of Balance* (an easy-to-read booklet on chronic pain issues, with cartoon drawings)

Klein & Sobel, *Backache Relief* (the results of a large survey of back pain patients)

Robin McKenzie, *Treat Your Own Back* (a guide to causes of back pain and specific exercise programs)

Melnick, Saunders & Saunders, *Managing Back Pain* (an easy-to-understand explanation of the effects of posture on the back, with recommended exercises)

Sefra Pitzele, *We Are Not Alone* (a book that explores the difficulties of living with chronic illness and offers practical help)

Cheri Register, *Living With Chronic Illness* (another personal view of chronic illness. Both Pitzele and Register are very helpful from an emotional standpoint.)

Duane Saunders, *The Back Care Program* (a practical and inexpensive guide for proper posture in all kinds of activities - a must!)

Duane Saunders, *For Your Neck* (a booklet on the effects of posture on neck pain, with recommended exercises)

Julie Zimmerman, *The Almanac of Back Pain Treatments* (an in depth examination of the entire range of traditional and alternative treatment approaches for back pain, including their pros and cons)

Julie Zimmerman, *Chronic Back Pain: Moving On* (an examination of the causes and effects of chronic pain and the range of treatment and management options for people living with chronic back problems)

Recommendations for Health Professionals

Back pain is often a difficult and frustrating condition to diagnose and treat. It is important to take the time to truly assess and evaluate your patient, relating symptoms to the patient's functional mobility and structural abnormalities. Apply the appropriate treatments based on your evaluation and then reevaluate to determine the patient's response to treatment. Health care practitioners who are irrevocably dedicated to one philosophy may not best serve the back pain patient. As one physical therapist writes, *"We cannot afford to be narrow-minded or isolated in our treatment procedures. As our people are varied, so too are their neuromusculoskeletal systems; we must treat them individually and thoroughly."* [2]

Patients need to be reassured that low back syndrome is not life-threatening and need the chance to ask questions and discuss their anxieties. Many don't know whether your treatment approach is symptomatic or curative; many assume that when their pain is reduced, the home program you recommended is no longer necessary. They need to understand that many of the most effective treatments for back pain require the patients to make permanent life-style changes, (e.g., posture, physical conditioning, exercise programs, common sense). It is in the interest of both practitioner and patient to work as a team, each with certain responsibilities. You don't have all the answers and should be able to admit that; the patient shouldn't expect to given a magic bullet.

It is a major challenge to create an individualized program out of the broad range of treatment options available for back problems. Part of your arsenal in combatting your patient's back pain is the ability to make appropriate referrals; an awareness of your limitations is the mark of a fine and effective health professional.

Recommended Reading

Diagnosis
- Kirkaldy-Willis, "A More Precise Diagnosis for Low Back Pain"
- Paris, "Physical Signs of Instability"
- Headley, "Postural Homeostasis"

Physicians & Pain Patients
- Cassel, "The Nature of Suffering and the Goals of Medicine"
- Cailliet, *Low Back Pain Syndrome*, 1988 edition

Indications for Surgery
- Fager, "Beware the Quick Fix for Back Pain"
- Fager, "Facts and Fallacies of Spinal Disorders: A Neurosurgeon's Viewpoint"

Chapter 14

Spondylosis
• Burkart & Beresford, "The Aging Intervertebral Disk"

Sacro-Iliac Joint Dysfunction
• Beal, "The Sacroiliac Problem: Review of Anatomy, Mechanics and Diagnosis"
• Bellamy, Park & Rooney, "What Do We Know About the Sacroiliac Joint"
• DonTigny, "Function and Pathomechanics of the Sacroiliac Joint"
• Grieve, "Lumbo-pelvic Rhythm and Mechanical Dysfunction of the Sacro-iliac Joint"

Exercise
• Jackson & Brown, "Analysis of Current Approaches and a Practical Guide to Prescription of Exercise"
• McGavin, "The McKenzie Approach to Spinal Pain"

Manipulation & Mobilization
• Consumer Reports Books, *Health Quackery*
• DiFabio, "Clinical Assessment of Manipulation and Mobilization of the Lumbar Spine"
• Paris, *The Spine* (course notes)

Overview of Musculoskeletal Dysfunction
• Kaplan & Tanner, *Musculoskeletal Pain and Disability*
• Kessler & Hertling, *Management of Common Musculoskeletal Disorders*
• Saunders, *Evaluation, Treatment and Prevention of Musculoskeletal Disorders*

Conclusion: Moving On

The Diagnosis and Misdiagnosis of Back Pain is concerned with the conditions which cause back pain and the professionals and procedures involved in diagnosing them. It attempts to give you, the back pain patient, enough information to understand the diagnostic possibilities you may be faced with and their rationales. The goal is to allow you to make informed decisions to help in the difficult task of finding the answers that will minimize your back pain. You may be one of the many people who will not receive a clear and accurate explanation for their symptoms; this doesn't mean you have to continue the search indefinitely. With or without a diagnosis, there are many treatment options available to help reduce your pain and dysfunc-

126

tion. When you have explored your options and made your choices, then relegate the pain to a less central place in your life. It's time to return to the essential task of making the best of your world and yourself!

Footnotes

1 Klein & Sobel, *Backache Relief*
2 David Reese, "Keep P.T. the Art That It Is"

Appendix A

Glossary

abduction - movement away from the midline of the body

active - performed through the effort of muscle contraction following nerve stimulation

acupressure - treatment approach using deep thumb or finger pressure on acupuncture points

acupuncture - treatment approach using needles inserted into the skin at points representing the body's meridians

acute - of recent onset; having a short, relatively severe course

acutherapy - acupuncture or acupressure

adduction - movement toward the midline of the body

adhesion - abnormal binding down of soft tissue

aerobics - exercise that increases the body's use of oxygen

ambulation - walking

ankylosing spondylitis - a form of arthritis, also called Marie Strumpel's disease

annulus fibrosis - the outer part of an intervertebral disk

anomaly - abnormality

antagonist - the muscle which performs movement in the opposite direction to the muscle being discussed

anterior - toward the front of the body

anterior dysfunction - displacement of the sacrum relative to the ilia, occurring on forward flexion

anterior superior iliac spine - bony landmark on the pelvis commonly called the "hip bone"

anterolateral - angled toward the front and side of the body

arachnoid - the middle of the three meninges

arthritis - a condition characterized by inflammation of the joints

articular - pertaining to a joint

articular cartilage - cartilaginous surface of a joint at the end of a bone

articular process - superior or inferior bony prominence of a vertebra which forms a facet joint with an adjacent vertebra

ASIS - see anterior superior iliac spine

asymptomatic - without symptoms; painless

atrophy - wasting or shrinking of muscle fibers

auto-immune - pertaining to conditions in which the body produces antibodies against its own tissues

autonomic nervous system - portion of the nervous system concerned with regulation of the heart muscle, smooth muscle and glands

back muscles - see spinal muscles

back school - a class offered by PT departments which teaches proper use of the spine

bedrest, total - bedrest during which any weight-bearing is eliminated or minimized

bilateral - involving both right and left sides of the body

biofeedback - a modality which visually or auditorally represents physiological responses of the body to enable patients to learn to consciously produce physical changes

body mechanics - the posture of the body in motion

bone - hard, immobile structure which makes up the skeleton or framework of the body

bone scan - radiographic test involving the injection of dye into a vein in order to identify diseases of bone

bone spur - abnormal growth of bony tissue often associated with degenerative changes

capsule - see joint capsule

cartilage - hard, structural tissue which makes up part of the skeleton; found at the ends of bones, ribs and joint surfaces

CAT scan - computerized axial tomography; a radiographic test which provides a three-dimensional picture of bone and soft tissue

catecholamines - compounds produced by the body in response to stress

cauda equina syndrome - a serious condition in which a nerve or nerves in the lower part of the spinal canal are compressed, causing bladder symptoms

central nervous system - the brain and spinal cord

cerebro-spinal fluid - a fluid produced by the brain which is contained between the meninges and which serves a shock-absorbing role for the central nervous system

cervical - pertaining to the neck region

cervical roll - cylindrical pillow placed behind the neck to maintain the cervical lordosis

chronic - long-lasting; pertaining to a medical condition lasting longer than three to six months

chronic pain syndrome - long-term pain which is reinforced by the environment and associated with a specific personality profile

coccyx - the vertebral segments comprising the tailbone

contract - shorten, referring to a muscle when stimulated

contraction - tensing or shortening of a muscle in response to a nerve stimulus

contraindicated - to be avoided; not recommended

contralateral - pertaining to the opposite side of the body

cortical bone - outer part of the shaft of a bone

cortisone - a hormone with anti-inflammatory properties

counterstrain - a technique which maintains the muscle in a relaxed, non-strained posture for 90 seconds

cranial - pertaining to the skull or head

craniosacral rhythm - the pulse produced by the cyclical production of CSF

CSF - see cerebro-spinal fluid

CT scan - see CAT scan

deafferation - the cutting of a sensory nerve

dermatome - skin area innervated by one spinal nerve

diathermy - machine which uses electricity to apply heat to surface tissues

differential diagnosis - the process of ruling out possible pathology to arrive at a definitive diagnosis

disc - see disk

disk - the structure located between the vertebral bodies, composed of a fibrous outer ring and an inner gelatin-like center

diskectomy - a surgical procedure to remove the disk or nucleus of the disk

disk fragment - extruded piece of the nucleus of the disk

diskography - a radiographic procedure in which dye is injected into a disk to identify a rupture

dislocation - total disruption of the opposing surfaces of a joint

DO - doctor of osteopathy

dural sheath (dura) - the outer covering of a nerve root

dura mater (dura) - the outermost of the three meninges which covers the brain and spinal cord
dysfunction - increased, decreased or abnormal movement

electromyography - diagnostic test in which needle electrodes inserted into muscle tissue relay
    electrical impulses from the muscle in order to identify nervous system diseases
electrotherapy - the therapeutic use of electricity
embryological - formed during the development of a fetus
EMG - see electromyography
endorphin - natural pain-killing substance produced by the body
endurance - lasting power; ability to maintain a position or perform numerous repetitions of a
    movement
ER - external rotation
erector spinae - back muscles which extend the trunk
ergonomics - adaptation of the workplace and equipment to accommodate an injured worker
extensibility - amount of stretch in a tissue
extension - motion of straightening a joint or body part
extensor muscles - see spinal muscles
external rotation - hip or shoulder movement in which the long bone of the thigh or arm rolls
    outward
extrusion - escaping of tissue outside its normal boundaries

facet joint - a synovial joint formed by the articular processes of two vertebrae
facilitation - see muscle facilitation
fascia - connective tissue of the body
femur - thigh bone
fiber - small segment of connective or muscle tissue; a nerve process
fibrillation - spontaneous contractions of individual muscle cells or fibers
fibromyalgia - see fibrositis
fibromyositis - see fibrositis
fibrositis - a condition characterized by diffuse tender areas of musculoskeletal tissues
flexion - motion of bending a joint or body part
function - use; movement
functional mobility - ability of the body to move normally to perform activities of daily living
functional restoration - work hardening
fusion - a surgical procedure in which bone fragments are inserted into an unstable joint to form
    a solid mass of bone

gate control theory - concept that pain sensations are blocked at the spinal cord by sensory
    stimulation
golfer's lift - stance incorporating extension of the non-weight bearing leg when bending forward
GP - general practitioner
gluteals - muscles at the back and sides of the pelvis which extend or abduct the hip
gluteal sets - tensing of the gluteus maximus muscles by squeezing the buttocks together

hamstrings - the muscles at the back of the thigh which extend the hip and flex the knee
herniated, herniation - see ruptured, rupture
holism - approach to health care which emphasizes the whole person
hyperextension - extension past a neutral trunk position
hypermobility - excessive movement of joints

hypomobility - below-average movement of joints
hypertonus - excessive amount of muscle tone

iatrogenic - caused by medical treatment
iliac crest - large curved portion of the upper pelvis, starting at what is commonly called the "hip bone"
ilium (pl. - ilia) - part of the pelvis which lies posterior and superior and forms a joint with the sacrum
impingement - compression, usually referring to a nerve root compression due to a disk rupture
inhibition - see muscle inhibition
innervation - nerve supply to a body part, usually referring to the nerve which stimulates a specific muscle
inominates - the joint surfaces of the pelvis which connect with the sacrum
internal rotation - a motion of the shoulder or hip joint in which the long bone of the upper arm or thigh rolls inward
interspinous ligaments - short ligaments connecting spinous processes of the vertebrae
intra-abdominal pressure - the tension of the contents of the abdomen against a contraction of the abdominal muscles
IR - internal rotation
internship - the year of hospital training following medical school
intervertebral - between the vertebrae
ischemia - decreased blood supply
ischium - part of the pelvis which lies posterior and inferior
isometrics - muscle contractions in which no joint movement occurs

joint - moveable part of the body's skeleton where the ends of two bones are joined
joint capsule - the sheath which surrounds and protects a synovial joint
joint play - small, involuntary movements in a joint in response to an outside force

kinesiology - the applied study of the principles and mechanics of movement
kinesiotherapy - a profession providing rehabilitation under the direction of physiatrist
KT - kinesiotherapist
kyphosis - convex curve of the spine, normal in the thoracic and sacral areas

lamina - the posterior part of the vertebral arch
laminectomy - surgical removal of the posterior arch of a vertebra, usually done to relieve nerve root compression from a ruptured disk
lateral flexion - movement of the neck or trunk to the side, away from the body's midline
lengthening contraction - tensing of a muscle to control movement in a direction opposite to its normal action
lesion - site of an injury
ligament - tough inelastic tissue which supports joints
longitudinal ligaments - long anterior and posterior ligaments running the length of the spinal column and connecting the vertebral bodies
long-sitting - sitting position with hips flexed and knees extended
lordosis - concave curve of the spine, normal in the cervical and lumbar areas
low back syndrome - vague diagnosis referring to non life-threatening conditions affecting the lumbo-sacral spine and its related structures
lumbago - common term for backache

lumbar - pertaining to the low back area

lumbar roll - approximately four-inch cylindrical pillow used to maintain a lumbar lordosis

magnetic resonance imaging - a non-invasive diagnostic test in which magnetic waves are used to image soft tissues

malingering - pretending to be ill

malleolus - ankle bone

manipulation - treatment approach in which the practitioner imparts a sudden thrust to realign body structures and/or reduce functional limitations

manual therapy - treatment in which the practitioner's hands are used to effect changes in the body

MD - medical doctor; one who has graduated from a four-year medical school

meninges - the three membranes which surround the brain and spinal cord

meniscus - crescent-shaped structure made up of cartilage and fibrous tissue which attaches to a joint capsule and extends into a joint

MENS - microcurrent therapy

meridian - one of 12 channels of vital energy in the body; a concept used in acupuncture

microcurrent therapy - form of electrotherapy which uses a current of low amperage to promote healing

mixers - chiropractors who use other treatment forms in addition to manipulation

mobilization - gentle form of manual therapy used to restore normal movement to body structures

MRI - magnetic resonance imaging

muscle - structure made up of elastic, contractile fibers which shortens when stimulated by a nerve to produce movement at a joint

muscle energy techniques - treatment which uses nervous system mechanisms to inhibit or facilitate a specific muscle

muscle facilitation - technique which uses nervous system mechanisms to increase muscle tone and stimulate a muscle to contract

muscle fatigue - technique using a strong contraction of a tight muscle to cause subsequent inhibition and relaxation of that muscle

muscle inhibition - use of nervous system mechanisms to reduce tone or spasm in tight muscles

muscle tone - see tone

myelogram - a radiographic test in which cerebro-spinal fluid is removed from the space surrounding the spinal cord and dye is injected in order to identify nerve root compression

myofascial - pertaining to the muscles and their surrounding connective tissue

myofascial pain syndrome - see fibrositis

nerve - a cell which transmits impulses within the nervous system to carry information to and from the brain or spinal cord; a bundle of nerve projections and their coverings

nerve root - part of the nervous system connecting the spinal cord and peripheral nerves which lies within the spinal canal

nerve root compression - pressure against a nerve root, commonly from a ruptured disk or bone spur, which produces pain and neurologic signs

neurological - neurologic

neurologic signs - symptoms which indicate involvement of the nervous system; with nerve root compression, numbness, weakness, decreased reflexes

neurology - a medical specialty which treats diseases of the nervous system

neurosurgery - a medical specialty where operations are performed on the nervous system or its surrounding structures nightshades - a category of foods which includes potatoes, tomatoes and tobacco

NMR - nuclear magnetic resonance (see MRI)

nociceptive - painful, injury producing

nucleus pulposis - the gelatin-like, water-binding center of an intervertebral disk

obliques - the two abdominal muscles which perform diagonal trunk flexion

occupational therapy - an allied medical profession concerned with functional activities for rehabilitation, developmental and psychiatric treatment

opposition - state in which body surfaces are in close proximity and parallel to each other, as with joint surfaces or thumb to finger pad

organic - physical; pertaining to the body

orthopedic - pertaining to the musculoskeletal system

orthopedic surgeon - an MD specializing in operations to correct conditions of the musculoskeletal system

orthopod - slang for orthopedic surgeon

osteoarthritis - condition characterized by localized degenerative changes in joints

osteophyte - bone spur

osteoporosis - abnormal thinning of the bones

osteopath - a graduate from a four-year school of osteopathic medicine with a DO degree

OT - occupational therapist or occupational therapy

pain behavior - actions and personality characteristics typical of patients whose chronic pain is reinforced by their environments

pain clinic - a rehabilitation center with a multidisciplinary approach to chronic pain

pain coping - therapeutic techniques to help chronic pain patients adjust to their disabilities

pain inhibition - techniques used to block the transmission of pain messages to the brain

pain management - therapeutic techniques to help chronic pain patients minimize their pain and maximize their function

palpation - examination by touch

paraspinal - in the area of the spine

paraspinal muscles - see spinal muscles

parasympathetic nervous system - the cranio-sacral portion of the autonomic nervous system

paravertebral - in the area of the vertebrae

paravertebral muscles - see spinal muscles

paresthesia - abnormal sensation, including pins-and-needles, tingling, burning

passive - performed by an outside force without active muscle contraction

pathology - diseased or abnormal state

pedicle - segment of the vertebral arch which joins the vertebral body to the lamina

pelvic obliquity - asymmetry of the pelvic ring creating a wind-blown effect

pelvic tilt - upward movement of the front of the pelvis which flattens the lumbar curve and which is accomplished by a contraction of the abdominal and gluteal muscles

pelvis - large bony ring joined to the spine at the sacrum and to the legs at the hip joints

perception - a person's knowledge of the physical world as interpreted by the brain

perianal - surrounding the anus

periosteum - outer covering of bone

peripheral - away from the central part of the body, usually referring to structures in the arms and legs

peripheral nervous system - the nerves of the body, peripheral to the spinal cord

perirectal - area surrounding the anus and end part of the rectum pharmacology - the study of drugs and their effects on the body

physiatrist - an MD specializing in physical medicine and non-surgical rehabilitation

physical therapy - an allied health profession which uses physical means to promote health and rehabilitation

pia mater - the innermost of the three meninges

piriformis - a muscle in the buttock through or under which the sciatic nerve passes

piriformis syndrome - a condition in which spasm of the piriformis muscle causes sciatic nerve compression

placebo - treatment which has no beneficial physical effects

placebo effect - relief of symptoms following the use of a placebo

posterior - toward the back of the body

posterior superior iliac spine - bony landmark on the pelvis near the top of the sacrum

posterolateral - angled toward the back and side of the body

post-op - following a surgical procedure

posture - the position one assumes against gravity

pre-op - preceding a surgical procedure

press-ups - an exercise of passive hyperextension in prone, used for disk prolapse

prognosis - outlook of an illness; chances for recovery

prolapsed disk - condition in which the nucleus of the disk pushes against the annular fibers, causing them to bulge into the spinal canal

proliferant - substance which stimulates the production of new tissue

prone - stomach-lying

protrusion - bulging of tissue beyond its normal boundary

PSIS - posterior superior iliac spine

psychiatrist - an MD specializing in treatment of emotional or mental problems

psychogenic - originating in the mind

PT - physical therapy or physical therapist

pubic symphysis - fibrous joint at the front of the pelvis

pubis - anterior part of the pelvis

pyriformis - see piriformis

Qi - Chinese concept meaning the body's vital energy

radiation - movement of symptoms from an injured area, often following the path of a nerve; electromagnetic waves

radicular - pertaining to a specific nerve root and its distribution

radiographic - pertaining to diagnostic tests in which x-rays or other electromagnetic waves are used to visualize internal parts of the body, including x-rays, CAT scans, MRI, myelograms, bone scans, etc.

radiologic/radiological - see radiographic

radiologist - an MD specializing in the performance and interpretation of radiographic testing

range of motion - the full arc of movement available at a joint

reciprocal inhibition - technique using a strong contraction of a tight muscle which causes subsequent inhibition and relaxation of that muscle

rectal tone - responsiveness of the sphincter muscles responsible for bowel retention

rectus - the abdominal muscle which performs straight trunk flexion

reflex - an immediate motor response following a sensory stimulus which initially bypasses the brain

reflex inhibition - reduction of muscle spasm through the use of nervous system mechanisms residency - hospital training for MDs or DOs following internship, for specialization

rheumatoid - pertaining to the joints of the body

ROM - see range of motion

rotation - twisting movement around a body axis

ruptured disk - a condition in which part of the nucleus of a disk has extruded through the outer annular fibers into the spinal canal

sacro-iliac joint - the connection between the pelvis and sacrum

sacro-iliac joint dysfunction - a syndrome in which the SI joint is subluxed, inflamed or painful

sacral - pertaining to the spinal region between the low back and tailbone

sacrum - five vertebrae located below the lumbar vertebrae which are fused into one bone

sciatica - pain which follows the path of the sciatic nerve down the back of the leg

sciatic nerve - large nerve composed of a bundle of nerve fibers from the lumbar and sacral parts of the spinal cord, which runs down the back of the thigh and innervates the posterior thigh, lower leg and foot

sclerotome - deep tissues which are innervated by the one spinal nerve

scoliosis - lateral curvature of the spine

secondary gains - benefits resulting from an illness

sensory stimulation - any input that sends messages about touch, temperature, vibration, movement, etc. through the sensory receptors to the central nervous system

sequestration - condition in which a fragment from the nucleus of a disk is loose in the spinal canal

sheath - outer covering of a nerve or muscle

SI - sacro-iliac

SIJ - sacro-iliac joint

SIJD - sacro-iliac joint dysfunction

SLR - straight leg raise

somatic - pertaining to the body

somatic dysfunction - term used in osteopathy to indicate a functional disorder of the musculos-keletal system

somatogenic - originating in the body

spasm - painful sustained contraction of a muscle in response to an injury to the muscle or to other nearby structures

specialist - an MD or DO who has completed a residency program in a specialty field

sphincter - muscle which allows retentive control of the bladder or bowel

spinal canal - the space within the vertebral column in which the spinal cord is located

spinal column - vertebral column; the bony spine

spinal cord - structure containing bundles of nerves which connects the brain and peripheral nervous system and which is enclosed by the spinal column

spinal muscles - four muscles composed of short fibers which originate and insert on the vertebrae and which extend and stabilize the spine

spinous process - posterior bony projection of a vertebra

spondylolysis - defect in the bony arch of a vertebra causing spinal instability

spondylolisthesis - bilateral defect of the bony arch of a vertebra with anterior slipping of the affected vertebral body

spondylosis - degenerative disease of the spine, with changes of vertebrae, joints and disks

sprain - injury or tearing of ligaments

stenosis - abnormal congenital or degenerative narrowing of the spinal canal

straight leg raise - a test for nerve root compression in which the hip is flexed with the knee extended; an exercise to stretch the hamstring muscle

straights - chiropractors who limit their practice to manipulation of the spinal column

strain - injury or tearing of muscle tissue

strain-counterstrain - a technique using passive positioning to reduce sensory input from soft tissues in order to reduce muscle tone

strength - the amount of resistance a muscle can overcome in a single repetition

structure - physical components of the body

subchondral bone - part of a bone located below the articular cartilage

subluxation - partial disruption of the opposing surfaces of a joint; slight vertebral malalignment

supine - back-lying

sympathetic nervous system - throacolumbar portion of the autonomic nervous system

symptom - a change in a patient's condition, indicating a dysfunctional state

syndrome - a set of symptoms which occur together, indicating a specific medical condition

synovial fluid - substance produced by the lining of a joint to provide shock-absorption, lubrication and protection for the joint

synovial joint - joint surrounded by a fluid-producing synovial membrane; a joint with a measurable amount of movement

synovial lining/membrane - the inner lining of a joint which secretes synovial fluid

systemic - affecting the whole body

tendon - non-elastic part of a muscle; inelastic cord which attaches a muscle to a bone

tendonitis - inflammation of a tendon

tenosynovitis - inflammation of a tendon and synovial membrane of a joint

TENS - see transcutaneous electrical nerve stimulation

therapeutic - beneficial; causing reversal of pathology or symptoms

thermograph - diagnostic tool which measures spinal heat

thoracic - pertaining to the trunk or to the part of the spine between the neck and waist

thrust - a sudden, high-velocity, low amplitude force applied to a specific structure of the body

tone - readiness of a muscle to contract; a muscle's resistance to stretch

total bedrest - see bedrest

toxic - poisonous to the body

traction - a pulling force which separates joint surfaces

transcutaneous electrical nerve stimulation - a modality which imparts a mild electrical current to the skin to inhibit pain elsewhere in the body

transverse ligaments - short ligaments connecting the transverse processes of two vertebrae

transverse process - bony lateral projection of a vertebra to which muscles and ligaments attach

trigger point - most tender spot in a muscle; tender area of fibrous bands in a muscle

trochanter - bony prominence on the femur

trochanteric belt - stabilizing support which surrounds the pelvis at hip level to provide support for the SI joint

tropism - degenerative scoliosis of individual spinal segments caused by asymmetry of disks or vertebrae

ultra-sound - machine which uses sound waves to produce heat in deep tissues

Valsalva maneuver - tightening of the abdominal muscles with a closed glottis; straining

vascular - having a large blood supply

vertebra - single bony segment of the spinal column

vertebrae - plural of vertebra

vertebral body - the largest part of a vertebra, separated from other vertebral bodies by disks

vertebral column - spinal column; bony spine

vertebral process - one of a number of bony projections of a vertebra

viscera - the large interior organs of the body

Williams flexion exercises - treatment regime for low back pain which emphasizes flexion postures and abdominal strengthening

work hardening - a treatment program which simulates a patient's work environment in order to return injured workers to the job safely and quickly

x-ray - a radiographic test in which the bones of the body are visualized

yin and yang - names for the Chinese concept of the two opposing influences on the body

Appendix B

Bibliography

Abraham, Edward, *Freedom from Back Pain: An Orthopedist's Self-Help Guide*, Rodale, 1986

Allen, Henry, "That Back's Gotta Come Out," *The Washington Post*, April 29, 1990

American Medical Association, *The American Medical Association Book of Back Care*, Random House, 1982

American Osteopathic Association, informational literature, 1987-1989

"Approaches to Musculoskeletal Problems: Focus on the Low Back," Robert M. True, M.D. Symposium, April 26-27, 1985, South Portland, Maine

Apts, David & Blankenship, Keith, *Back Facts for the American Back School*, FPR, Inc., 1981

The Back Letter, "Memo on Body Mechanics," Ed. Theresa Reger, Skol Publishing

The Back Letter, Ed. Theresa Reger, Skol Publishing, Vol. 4, No. 2-9, December 1989-July, 1990

Barnes, John, "Benefits of Myofascial Release, Craniosacral Therapy Explained," *Physical Therapy Forum*, Aug., 29, 1984

Barnes, John, "Pro: Never Trademarked Myofascial Release," *P.T. Bulletin*, Feb. 17, 1988

Barnes, John, "Therapeutic Insight," *Physical Therapy Forum*, June 25, 1986

Batson, Glenna, "Reeducating or Strengthening: Relooking at the Pelvic Tilt," *Physical Therapy Forum*, Oct. 2, 1985

Beal, Myron, "The Sacroiliac Problem: Review of Anatomy, Mechanics and Diagnosis," *Journal of Amer. Osteopathic Assoc.*, Vol. 81, No. 10, June, 1982

Bellamy, Nicholas, Park, William & Rooney, Patrick, "What Do We Know About the Sacroiliac Joint," *Seminars in Arthritis and Rheumatism*, Vol. 12, No. 3, February, 1983

Benanti, Joseph & Ellis, Jeffrey, "Holistic Medicine a 'Crisis' for PTs," *PT Bulletin*, Jan. 18, 1989

Benjamin, Ben, "The Mystery of Lower Back Pain," Parts I & II, *Massage Therapy Journal*, Fall 1988 & Winter 1989

Blackburn, Stan & Portney, Leslie Gross, "Electromyographic Activity of Back Musculature During Williams' Flexion Exercises," Physical Therapy, Vol. 61, No. 6, June, 1981

Brena, Steven F., *Chronic Pain: America's Hidden Epidemic*, Atheneum/SMI, 1978

Bunch, Richard, "Con: Myofascial Release Traced Back Decades," *P.T. Bulletin*, Feb. 17, 1988

Burkart, Sandy & Beresford, William, "The Aging Intervertebral Disk," *Physical Therapy*, Vol. 59, No. 8, August, 1979

Cailliet, Rene, *Low Back Pain Syndrome*, Second Edition, F.A. Davis, 1962

Cailliet, Rene, *Low Back Pain Syndrome*, Edition 4, F.A. Davis, 1988

Caplan, Deborah, *Back Trouble*, Triad Publishing Co., 1987

Carmichael, Joel, "Inter- and Intra-Examiner Reliability of Palpation for Sacroiliac Joint Dysfunction," *Journal of Manipulative and Physiological Therapeutics*, Vol. 10, No. 4, August, 1987

Carper, Jean, *Health Care U.S.A.*, Prentice Hall Press, 1987

Carr, Sharon & Phillips, Cathy L., "Helping TMJ Patients to Help Themselves," *Physical Therapy Forum*, Jan. 8, 1990

Carroll, Sarah, "Hypnosis: An Underutilized Modality," *Physical Therapy Forum*

Carter, Mildred, *Helping Yourself With Foot Reflexology*, Parker Publishing Co., 1969

Cassel, Eric, "The Nature of Suffering and the Goals of Medicine," *New England Journal of Medicine*, Vol. 306, No. 11, March 18, 1982

Chapman-Smith, David, "Chiropractic – A Referenced Source of Modern Concepts, New Evidence," Practice Makers Products Inc., 1988

CIBA Clinical Symposia,"Low Back Pain," Vol. 25, Number 3, CIBA Pharmaceutical Co., 1973

Cibulka, Michael & Koldehoff, Rhonda, "Evaluating Chronic Sacroiliac Joint Dysfunction," *Clinical Management*, Vol. 6, No. 4, 1987

Cibulka, Michael & Koldehoff, Rhonda, "Leg Length Disparity and Its Effect on Sacroiliac Joint Dysfunction," *Clinical Management*, Vol. 6, No. 5, 1987

Colbin, Annemarie, *Food and Healing*, Ballantine Books, 1986

Consumer Reports Books, Editors of, *Health Quackery: Consumers Union's Report on False Health Claims, Worthless Remedies and Unproved Therapies*, Holt, Rhinehart and Winston, 1980

Cousins, Norman, *Anatomy of an Illness*, W.W. Norton & Co., 1979

Croce, Pat, "Put Stress to Rest," *Physical Therapy Forum*, August 21, 1989

Cuckler, John, Bernini, Philip, Wiesel, Sam, Booth, Robert, Ruthman, Richard & Pickens, Gary, "The Use of Epidural Steroids in the Treatment of Lumbar Radicular Pain," *The Journal of Bone & Joint Surgery*, Vol. 67-A, No. 1, January, 1985

Cyriax, James, *Textbook of Orthopaedic Medicine*, Baillier-Tindall, 1980

Derebery, Jane & Tullis, William, "Delayed Recovery in the Patient with a Work Compensable Injury," *Journal of Occupational Medicine*, Nov., 1983

Deyo, Richard, "Conservative Therapy for Low Back Pain," *JAMA*, Aug. 26, 1983, Vol. 250

Deyo, Richard, Loeser, John & Bigos, Stanley, "Herniated Lumbar Intervertebral Disk," *Annals of Internal Medicine*, Vol. 112, No. 8, April 15, 1990

Deyo, Richard, Walsh, Nicholas, Martin, Donald, Schoenfeld, Lawrence & Ramamurthy, Somayaji, "A Controlled Trial of Transcutaneous Electrical Nerve Stimulation (TENS) and Exercise for Chronic Low Back Pain," *The New England Journal of Medicine*, Vol. 322, No. 23, June 7, 1990

DiFabio, Richard, "Clinical Assessment of Manipulation and Mobilization of the Lumbar Spine," *Physical Therapy*, Vol. 66, No. 1, Jan., 1986

Dimick, Terry, "Kinesiotherapist Responds," *P.T. Bulletin*, July 4, 1990

Dommerholt, Jan, "Meridian Therapy – A New European Concept," *Physical Therapy Forum*, March 5, 1990

DonTigny, Richard, "Dysfunction of the Sacroiliac Joint and Its Treatment," *The Journal of Orthopaedic and Sports Medicine Therapy*, Vol. 1, No. 1, Summer, 1979

DonTingy, Richard, "Function and Pathomechanics of the Sacroiliac Joint," *Physical Therapy*, Vol. 65, No. 1, Jan., 1985

Edgelow, Peter, "Physical Examination of the Lumbosacral Complex," *Physical Therapy*, Vol. 59, No. 8, Aug., 1979

Elgee, Neil, "Norman Cousins' Sick Laughter Redux," *Archives of Internal Medicine*, Vol. 150, August, 1990

Fager, Charles, "Beware the Quick Fix for Back Pain," *Trends in Rehabilitation*, Winter, 1986

Fager, Charles, "Facts and Fallacies of Spinal Disorders: A Neurosurgeon's Viewpoint," *Evaluation and Treatment of Chronic Pain*

Fager, Charles, "The Neurosurgical Management of Lumbar Spine Disease," *New Developments in Medicine*, Vol. 3, No. 2, Sept., 1988

Fahey, Brian, "The Principles of Structural Diagnosis," *Physical Therapy Forum*, Oct. 23, 1989

Folan, Lilias, *Lilias Yoga and You*, Bantum Books, 1972

Friedman, Nancy, "Back Exercises for a Healthy Back," Krames Communications, 1985

Gildenberg, Philip L. & DeVaul, Richard A., *The Chronic Pain Patient*, Kargen, 1985

Glade, Phyllis, *Crystal Healing: The Next Step*, Llewellyn Publications, 1989

Glisan, Billy, Stith, William & Kiser, Sanford, "Physiology of Active Exercise in Rehabilitation of Back Injuries," *Health Tracks*, Vol. 2, Issue 1

Goering, Gail, "Treat Injured Workers Like Athletes," *P.T. Bulletin*, May 9, 1990

Gottlieb, Harold, Alperson, Burton, Koller, Reuben & Hockersmith, Virgil, "An Innovative Program for the Restoration of Patients with Chronic Back Pain," *Physical Therapy*, Vol. 59, No. 8, August, 1979

Grieve, Elizabeth "Lumbo-pelvic Rhythm and Mechanical Dysfunction of the Sacro-iliac Joint," *Physiotherapy*, Vol. 67, No. 6, June, 1981

Hay, Louise, *You Can Heal Your Life*, Hay House, 1984

Headley, Barbara, *Chronic Pain: Life Out of Balance*, H. Duane Saunders, 1987

Headley, Barbara, "Dynamic Stabilization," *Physical Therapy Forum*, June 4, 1990

Headley, Barbara, "Pain Vs. Suffering," *Physical Therapy Forum*, May 16, 1988

Headley, Barbara, "Postural Homeostasis," *Physical Therapy Forum*, Sept. 17, 1990

Hebert, Lauren, *Sex and Back Pain*, H. Duane Saunders, 1987

Heinrich, Steve, "Body Watch: The Importance of Dialogue and Myofascial Unwinding in Creating a Safe Place to Heal," *Physical Therapy Forum*, Feb. 5, 1990

Heller, Joseph & Hanson, Jan, *The Client's Handbook*, The Body of Knowledge, Mt. Shasta, Ca.

Horwich, Mark, "Low Back Pain: The Neurologist's View," *Drug Therapy*, Dec., 1982

Hutchinson, Lynn, "Direct Access and Preventative Therapy," *Physical Therapy Forum*, Sept., 25, 1989

Imrie, David, *Goodbye Back Ache*, Prentice-Hall/Newcastle, 1983

Irwin, Yukiko, *Shiatzu*, J.B. Lippincott, 1976

Ishmael, William & Shorbe, Howard, "Care of the Back," J.B. Lippincott Co., 1953

Jackson, Claudia & Brown, Mark, "Analysis of Current Approaches and a Practical Guide to Prescription of Exercise," *Clinical Orthopaedics*, No. 179, October, 1983

Jackson, Claudia & Brown, Mark, "Is There a Role for Exercise in the Treatments of Patients with Low Back Pain," *Clinical Orthopaedics*, No. 179, October, 1983

Jacobs, Bernard, "Low Back Pain: The Orthopedist's View," *Drug Therapy*, Dec., 1982

Jones, Bob, *The Difference a D.O. Makes*, Osteopathic Medicine in the Twentieth Century, Times-Journal Publishing Co., Oklahoma City, Ok., 1978

Jones, Frank Pierce, *Body Awareness in Action: A Study of the Alexander Technique*, Schocken Books, 1979

Kaplan, Paul & Tanner, Ellen, *Musculoskeletal Pain and Disability*, Appleton & Lange, 1989

Kessler, Randolph, "Acute Symptomatic Disk Prolapse," *Physical Therapy*, Vol. 59, No. 8, Aug., 1979

Kessler, Randolph & Hertling, Darlene, *Management of Common Musculoskeletal Disorders*,

Harper & Row, 1983

Kim, Nini, "Holistic Medicine Requires Different World View," *PT Bulletin*, March 1, 1989

Kirkaldy-Willis, W.H., *Managing Low Back Pain*, Churchill Livingstone, 1988

Kirkaldy-Willis, W.H. & Hill, R.J., "A More Precise Diagnosis for Low Back Pain," *Spine*, Vol. 4, No. 2, Mar./Apr., 1979

Klein, Arthur & Sobel, Dava, *Backache Relief*, New American Library, 1985

Knott, Margaret & Voss, Dorothy, *Proprioceptive Neuramuscular Facilitation*, Harper & Row, 1968

Kotzsch, Ronald, "AIDS: Putting an Alternative to the Test," *East West*, Sept., 1986

Krumhansl, Bernice & Nowacek, Charles, "Case Study – Spinal Manipulation Under Anaesthesia," *Physical Therapy Forum*, Sept. 4, 1989

Lamb, David, "The Neurology of Spinal Pain," *Physical Therapy*, Vol. 59, No. 8, Aug., 1979

Langone, John, *Chiropractors: A Consumer's Guide*, Addison-Wesley Publicling Co., 1982

Lauterback, Joyce, "The Mind-Body Connection – Is There More?" *Physical Therapy Forum*, July 17, 1989

Lawn, George, "How to Lift – Is There a Right Way?" *Physical Therapy Forum*, June 12, 1985

Lehman, Betsy, "Feeling Bad About Feeling Bad," *The Good Health Magazine (Boston Globe)*, October 8, 1989

Levine, David B., *The Painful Low Back*, Merck, Sharp & Dohme, 1979

Lewith, Geroge & Horn, Sandra, *Drug Free Pain Relief*, Thorsons Publishers, 1987

Lockett, Ricky, "Pyriformis Syndrome – Diagnosis and Treatment," *Physical Therapy Forum*, Aug. 22, 1988

MacPhee, Patricia, "Chronic Pain and the Role of Occupational Therapy," *Physical Therapy Forum*, Sept. 18, 1989

Maitland, G.D., *Vertebral Manipulation*, Butterworths, 1977

Marantz, Steve, "The Perfect Chair," *The Boston Globe*, Oct. 8, 1989

Mayer, Tom, "Rehabilitation of the Patient with Spinal Pain," *The Orthopedic Clinics of North America*, Vol. 14, No. 3, July 1983

McGavin, James, "The McKenzie Approach to Spinal Pain," *Physical Therapy Forum*, July 5, 1988

McKenzie, Robin, *Treat Your Own Back*, Spinal Publications Ltd., 1985

McGregor, Marion & Cassidy, David, "Post-surgical Sacroiliac Joint Syndrome," *Journal of Manipulative and Physiologic Therapeutics*, Vol. 6, No. 1, March, 1983

Mead, Mark, "Chiropractic's New Wave," *East West*, November, 1989

Melnick, Michael, Saunders, Robin & Saunders, Duane, *Managing Back Pain*, H. Duane Saunders, 1989

Miller, David, "Comparison of Electromyographic Activity in the Lumbar Paraspinal Muscles of Subjects with and without Low Back Pain," *Physical Therapy*, Vol. 65, No. 9, Sept., 1985

Mills, Simon & Finando, Steven, *Alternatives in Healing: An Open-Minded Approach to Finding the Best Treatment for Your Health Problems*, New American Library, 1989

Mixter, Jason, "Rolfing," (Editors) Lowe & Nechas, *Whole Body Healing*, Rodale Press, 1983

Montgomery, Edith, "Folsom Physical Therapy – A Different Approach to Back Rehabilitation," *Physical Therapy Forum*, June 13, 1988

Olsen, Paulette, "Body Mechanics Education – A Legacy for our Children," *Physical Therapy Forum*, April 23, 1990

Olsen, Paulette, "Brief Media Presentations on Back Care," *Physical Therapy Forum*, Nov. 27, 1989

Ondricek, Jana, "Techniques for Effective Therapeutic Management of Workmen's Compensation Patients," *Physical Therapy Forum*, April 30, 1990

Ongley, Milne, Klein, Robert, Dorman, Thomas, Eek, Bjom, & Hubert, Lawrence, "A New Approach to the Treatment of Chronic Back Pain," *The Lancet*, July 18, 1987

Paris, Stanley, "Anatomy as Related to Function and Pain," *The Orthopedic Clinics of North America*, Vol. 14, No. 3, July, 1983

Paris, Stanley, "Mobilization of the Spine," *Physical Therapy*, Vol. 59, No. 8, Aug., 1979

Paris, Stanley, "Physical Signs of Instability," *Spine*, Vol. 10, No. 3, 1985

Paris, Stanley, *The Spine*, (Course Notes), Stanley Paris, 1979

Picker, Robert, "Microcurrent Therapy: 'Jump-Starting' Healing with Bioelectricity," *Physical Therapy Forum*, June 10, 1989

Pitzele, Sefra Korbin, *We Are Not Alone: Learning to Live with Chronic Illness*, Workman Publishing, 1985

Potter, Nancy & Rothstein, Jules, "Intertester Reliability for Selected Clinical Tests of the Sacroiliac Joint," *Physical Therapy*, Vol. 65, No. 11, Nov., 1985

Prudden, Bonnie, *Pain Erasure*, Ballantine Books, 1980

P.T. Bulletin, "Benefits of 'Humor Therapy' Promoted," April 25, 1980

P.T. Bulletin, "Reactions Mixed to Back Surgery Alternative," August 30, 1989

Rashbaum, Ralph, "Radiofrequency Facet Denervation," *The Orthopedic Clinics of North America*, Vol. 14, No. 3, July, 1983

Reese, David, "Keep PT the Art That It Is," *P.T. Bulletin*, April 25, 1990

Register, Cheri, *Living with Chronic Illness: Days of Patience and Passion*, The Free Press (Maacmillan), 1987

Reuben, Carolyn, "AIDS: The Promise of Alternative Treatments," *East West*, Sept., 1986

Rice, John, Allen, Nancy & Caldwell, David, "Low Back Pain: The Rheumatologist's View," *Drug Therapy*, Dec., 1982

Richardson, Nancy, "Aston-Patterning," *Physical Therapy Forum*, Oct., 28, 1987

Rolf, Ida, "Structural Integration," *Confin. Psychiat.* 16, 1973

Samo, John, *Mind Over Back Pain*, Berkley Books, 1982

Saunders, H. Duane, *The Back Care Program*, H. Duane Saunders, 1983

Saunders, H. Duane, *Evaluation, Treatment and Prevention of Musculoskeletal Disorders*, H. Duane Saunders, 1985

Saunders, Duane, *For Your Neck*, H. Duane Saunders, 1986

Shapiro, Gary, "Ceasing the Struggle," *Physical Therapy Forum*, May 7, 1990

Shea, Michael, "MFR and the Psychosomatic Body," *Physical Therapy Forum*, April 23, 1990

Sherman, Carl, "The Medicolegal Thicket of Low Back Disability," *Aches and Pains*, April, 1982

Siegel, Bernie S., *Peace, Love and Healing*, Harper & Row, 1989

Simons, David & Travell, Janet, "Myofascial Origins of Low Back Pain," Parts 1-3, *Postgraduate Medicine*, Vol. 73, No. 2, Feb., 1983

Smith, Ralph Lee, *At Your Own Risk: The Case Against Chiropractic*, Trident Press, 1969

Solet, Jo, "Low Back Pain – An Overview," *Physical Therapy Forum*, August 7, 1989

Steer, Allen, Hardin, John & Malawista, Stephen, "Lyme Arthritis: A New Clinical Entity," *Hospital Practice*, April, 1978

Sternbach, Richard A., *Pain Patients; Traits and Treatments*, Academic Press, 1974

Stickland, Ellen, "Trouble with KTs," *PT Bulletin*

Tamayo, Rey, "Work Hardening – A Different Treatment Approach," *Physical Therapy Forum*, Feb. 26, 1990

Thomas, Lynn, Hislop, Helen & Waters, Robert, "Physiological Work Performance in Chronic Low Back Disability," *Physical Therapy*, Vol. 60, No. 4, April, 1980

Wallnofer, Heinrich & vonRottauscher, Anna, *Chinese Folk Medicine and Acupuncture*, Bell Publishing Co., 1965

Weiselfish, Sharon & Kain, Jay, "Introduction of Developmental Manual Therapy – An Integrated System Approach for Structural and Functional Rehabilitation," *Physical Therapy Forum*, Feb. 12, 1990

White, Arthur, "Injection Techniques for the Diagnosis and Treatment of Low Back Pain," *The Orthopedic Clinics of North America*, Vol. 14, No. 3, July, 1983

Wildman, Frank, "The Feldenkrais Method: Clinical Applications," *P.T. Forum*, Feb. 19, 1986

Wildman, Frank, "Learning – The Missing Link in Physical Therapy," *P.T. Forum*, Feb. 8, 1988

Wildman, Frank, "Training in the Feldenkrais Method," The Institute for Movement Studies, Berkeley, Ca.

Wilk, Chester, *Chiropractic Speaks Out*, Wilk Publishing Co., 1973

Willis, Judith, "Back Pain: Ubiquitous, Controversial," *FDA Consumer*, November, 1983

Wolf, Barbara, *Living With Pain*, The Seabury Press, 1977

Woodworth, Barbara, "Therapeutic Values of Tai Chi," *Physical Therapy Forum*, July 23, 1990

Wyatt, William, DO, literature for patients, 1987

Yunus, Muhammed, Masi, Alfonse, Calabro, John & Shah, Indravadan, "Primary Fibromyalgia," *Amer. Fam. Phys.*, May, 1982

Zacharkow, Dennis, "The Problems with Lumbar Support," *Physical Therapy Forum*, Sept. 10, 1990

Zimmerman, Julie, *Goals and Objectives for Developing Normal Movement Patterns*, Aspen, 1988

Zinman, David, "Focus on Back Pain," *Newsday*, Jan. 30, 1990

Index - The Diagnosis and Misdiagnosis of Back Pain

conservative treatment 29, 74

controversy surrounding back pain 6-9, 60, 71, 82, 85-6, 90-1, 103, 108, 121-2

cost of back pain 6

counseling 123

craniosacral therapy 92

curves of spine (see spinal curves)

degenerative changes/disease (see spondylosis)

diagnosis, chiropractic d 35-7, 44.; d. of dysfunction 30; diagnostic examination 53-5; diagnostic tests 49-53 [Fig. 5-1]; differential d. 44, 53-5, 57-63; difficulty/inability establishing firm d. 6-10, 28, 40, 44, 121, 126; individualization of d. 30, 44-5, 121-3, 124-5; osteopathic d. 34, 44; patient's role in d. 10, 122; referral for d. 27-9, 45, 125 (see misdiagnosis)

diathermy (see heat)

diskectomy (see surgery)

diskography 51

disks 15, 50, 95, 97 [Fig. 1-3, 1-5, 1-6, 1-7]; prolapsed/ruptured d.s 50-3, 59-63, 65-70 [Fig. 7-2, 7-3, 7-4]; treatment 71-4

doctors (see medical doctors)

driving 118

drugs (see medications)

dysfunction 29; diagnosis of d. 30; somatic d. 34-5

dura 67, 70 (see meninges)

electromyography 53, 91

EMG (see electromyography)

emotional/psychological factors, e./p. effects of pain 9, 44; e./p. f.s contributing to pain 44-5, 123 (see tension)

endorphins 24-5, 40

endurance 92

energy flow 45-6, 92

epiduralgram 53

epidural injection (see injection)

epiduralvenogram 53

equipment, seating 72, 118-20 [Fig. 13-2]

erector spinae 88-91 [Fig. 9-1]

exercise (see physical conditioning)

exercises, extension e.s 72, 92; flexibility e.s 91-2, 99; flexion e.s 30, 91-2; for disk prolapse 72 [Fig. 7-5]; for SIJD 108; individualization of e.s 30, 72, 122; relaxation e.s 92; strengthening e.s 92, 108

extension 22, 88, 90

facet joints 15, 21-2, 77, 80 [Fig. 1-6, 1-7, 1-8]; f.j. dysfunction 36, 51, 80-2, 95-8 [Fig. 8-4]; treatment 39-40, 80, 82, 99

family doctors 27-9, 43-5

fascia 21, 46, 59, 86-7, 92

feelings (see attitude; emotional/psych. factors)

fibrositis 87

financial cost of back pain 6

flexibility (see exercises, flex.; range of motion)

lumbar spine 13 [Fig. 1-1]; l. support [Fig. 13-2]
lying down (see bedrest)

magnetic resonance imaging 50-1, 74
malalignment (see asymmetry; dysfunction; subluxation)
manipulation 123; criticism of m. 40-1; chiropractic m. 35-40, 44; for diagnosis 62, 81; for disk
    dysfunction 71-2; for facet jnt. dysf. 82; for SIJD 107-8; osteopathic m. 33-5, 40, 44
manual therapy (see manipulation; mobilization)
massage 92-3, 113
McKenzie exercises 30 (see exercises for disk prolapse)
mechanical supports for sacro-iliac joint dysf. 108
medical doctors 27-9, 33, 43-5
medications 123
meninges 21
meniscus 15, 77 [Fig. 1-8C]; pinching of 80, 82
misdiagnosis 6, 8
Mixers 37
mobilization 30, 41, 123; for disk dysfunction 71; for facet jnt dysf. 82; for spondylosis 99
movement 15, 21-2, 88, 90; of sacro-iliac joint 101, 103-4
movement dysfunction (see dysfunction)
MRI (see magnetic resonance imaging)
muscles 15, 21-2, 88-90 [Fig. 9-1]; m. weakness 85, 90-3, 111; m.s & aging 97, 117; piriformis
    m. 111; strain/spasm 59-63, 85-7, 90-1; treatment 91-3, 113; (see abdominals; exercises;
    gluteals; hamstrings; spinal muscles; tension)
myelograms 51, 58, 74, 98 [Fig. 5-1]
myofascia/myofascial dysfunction (see fascia)
myofascial release 92

National Back Fitness Test 93
neck 63 [Fig. 1-1]; n. posture 118, 120 [Fig. 13-1]
nerve roots 21 [Fig. 1-3]; n.r. compression 51, 53, 59-62, 67-70, 99 [Fig. 7-4]; sacral n.r.c. 71
nervous system 21-2, 34-6, 38 [Fig. 1-3, 1-9]; pinching/entrapment of spinal n.s 36, 38, 81 [Fig.
    8-4]
neurological signs 62, 67, 69-70, 71-2, 74, 99
neurologists 28
neurosurgeons 28
nucleus pulposis (see disks)

obesity (see weight & back pain)
occupational therapists/therapy 30
orthopedic surgeons 28
osteopathy 33-5, 39-40, 43-5
osteoporosis 58, 97

pain 22-5; treatment 30, 40, 99; (see chronic pain)
pain-killers (see injections; medications)
pelvic tilts 91, 117-8, 123
pelvis 15, 111 [Fig. 1-2]
perception of pain 21-5, 40

physiatrists 28, 30, 44, 122
physical conditioning 124
physical exam 53-6
physical fitness instructors 122
physical limits (see balancing rest/activity)
physical therapists/therapy 29-30, 44, 122
physicians (see medical d.s; osteopaths)
piriformis muscle 60, 108, 111 [Fig. 12-1]
piriformis syndrome 60-3, 104, 111, 113-4
placebo effect 24-5, 40
positioning 118, 120, 123
positive attitude (see attitude)
posterior longitudinal ligaments (see longitudinal lig.s)
posture/body mechanics 60, 85, 92, 99, 115-20, 124 [Fig. 13-1, 13-2, 13-3]
press-ups 72 [Fig. 7-5]
prevalence of back pain 6
prevention of back pain 34, 38, 117
prolapse, disk (see disk)
psychiatrists/psychiatry 28
psychogenic pain 44, 59
psychotherapy (see counseling)
pubic symphysis 15 [Fig. 1-2]
pubis 15 [Fig. 1-2]

radiation of symptoms 60-1, 67, 69-71
radiographic tests 49-53, 60, 74, 81, 98 [Fig. 5-1]
radiologic tests (see radiographic tests)
range of motion 21-2, 86, 91-3, 97, 99, 117 (see hypomobility of jnt.s)
referral of patients 27-9, 39, 45, 125
referred pain 58-9, 69, 87, 98, 101, 113 (see radiation of symptoms)
reflexes 21
relaxation techniques 92-3, 123
residency 27
responsibility of patient 9-10, 45, 117, 122-4, 126-7
rest (see balance of rest/activity; bedrest)
rheumatologists 28
risks of treatment 8, 37-9, 40-1, 74, 107
rotation 22, 80
rupture, disk (see disks)

sacro-iliac joint 15, 60, 101-4, 113 [Fig. 1-2]
sacro-iliac joint dysfunction 30, 60-2, 103-9, 111; treatment 107-8
sacrum 13, 15 [Fig. 1-1, 1-2]; movement of s. 103-4; support in sitting [Fig. 13-2]
sciatica 69, 98, 113 (see nerve root compression; radiation of symptoms)
sciatic nerve [Fig. 12-1]; compression of 60, 111, 113
self-healing 34, 36, 45
sensation 21
sensory stimulation (see gate control theory)
sex 120

SIJ (see sacro-iliac joint)

sitting 67, 72, 98, 118, 120; supports for s. [Fig. 13-2]

society's view of disabilities 123

soft tissue 15, 21; s.t. dysfunction 59, 61-2, 82; (see muscles; ligaments; joint capsules; fascia)

somatic dysfunction 34-5, 44

spasm (see muscle spasm)

specializing physicians 28

spinal adjustment (see chiropractic manipulation)

spinal canal 21 [Fig. 1-4, 1-9]

spinal column 13, 15 [Fig. 1-1]

spinal cord 21 [Fig. 1-3, 1-9]

spinal curves 13, 97, 115-8 [Fig. 1-1, 13-1]

spinal muscles 15, 21-2, 88-90, 97, 115, 117 [Fig. 9-1]

spiritual healing 45-6

spondylosis 50, 59-62, 80, 95-9 [Fig. 10-1]; treatment 99

sports medicine 122

sprain (see ligament)

statistics on back pain 6-9, 43-4

stenosis 50-1, 58, 97-9

straight leg raise 62, 70, 81, 106, 113

Straights 36-7

strain (see muscle)

strength 15, 21, 88, 90, 92

stress (see tension)

stretching 91-2, 108, 113 (see exercises, flexibility; range of motion)

structural asymmetry (see asymmetry)

subluxation 36-9, 44, 80, 103 (see facet joint dysfunction, SIJ dysfunc.)

supports (see equipment, seating)

surgery 45-6, 74-5, 99, 113, 123

survey of back pain people 43-4

synovial joints 15, 77, 80, 103 [Fig. 1-8C]

synovial membrane 15 [Fig. 1-8 C]; pinching of 80

symptomatic treatment 28-9, 99

symptoms, of disk dysfunction 67, 69; of facet dysf. 81; of muscle strain/spasm 87; of piriformis syndrome 113; of SIJD 105-6; of spondylosis 98

tendons 21 [Fig. 1-8]

tension, emotional/muscle 44, 85, 92, 123

therapy (see physical t.; occupational t.; kinesiot.)

thermography 36, 50

thoracic spine 13 [Fig. 1-1]; t. support [Fig. 13-2]

thrust (see manipulation)

trauma 58, 67, 80, 85, 104, 111, 117

treatment, goals of 9-10, 62 (see t. for disk dysfunction, facet dysf., muscle dysf. spondylosis, SIJD, piriformis synd.)

trigger points 86-7, 93, 113

tumors 51, 58

ultrasound (see heat)

vertebra (pl. -ae) 13, 15, 77, 95-8 [Fig. 1-1, 1-3, 1-4, 1-5, 1-6, 1-7, 1-9]
vertebral bodies 13, 15, 95-8 [Fig. 1-4, 1-5, 1-6, 1-7]
vertebral column (see spinal column)
Veterans hospitals 30-1
visualization 92

weakness (see muscle w.)
weight & back pain 86, 118
Williams flexion exercises (see exercises, flexion)
work hardening 30, 123
work injuries 30, 123
worker's compensation 6

x-rays 28, 36-9, 50, 53, 95, 97-8, 101

yoga 92, 122

The Almanac of Back Pain Treatments

A complete guide to the rationales, benefits and risks of the traditional and alternative treatments for bad backs, by Julie Zimmerman, PT.

Table of Contents

Chronic Back Pain: Moving On

A complete guide to the treatment and management options for people living with bad backs, by Julie Zimmerman, PT.

Table of Contents

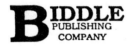

Order Form

Please send

_____ copies of *The Diagnosis and Misdiagnosis of Back Pain* at $9.95 each $ _____

_____ copies of *The Almanac of Back Pain Treatments* at $9.95 each $ _____

_____ copies of *Chronic Back Pain: Moving On* at $9.95 each $ _____

                             Subtotal $ _____

For orders of 3-5 books, deduct 15%
For orders of 6 or more books, deduct 20%.   − _____

Sales in state of Maine, add 5% sales tax.   + _____

Shipping, add $1.75 for first book, and $.75 for
each additional book.   + _____

                Total enclosed $ _____

Send check payable to: Biddle Publishing Company
                             Box 1305 - #103
                             Brunswick, Maine 04011

Expect up to four weeks for delivery.

For inquiries regarding discounts on larger orders, call 207-833-5016.